HEALTHY VEGAN 2022

DELICIOUS RECIPES TO CLEANSE YOUR BODY

GIGLIOLA URONI

Table of Contents

Spaghetti with Chorizo and Kidney Beans

INGREDIENTS

1 red onion, medium chopped

1 green bell pepper chopped

15 ounce can kidney beans

15 ounce can great northern beans

28 ounce crushed tomatoes

1/4 cup vegan chorizos, coarsely chopped

1 tsp. dried thyme

½ teaspoon salt

1/8 teaspoon black pepper

2 cups vegetable stock

8 ounces spaghetti noodles uncooked

1 ½ cups Vegan Cheese (Tofu Based)

Garnishing ingredients:

chopped green onions for serving

Put all of the ingredients except for pasta, vegan cheese, and garnishing ingredients in your slow cooker.

Combine and cover.

Cook on high heat for 4 hours or low heat for 7 hours.

Add the pasta and cooking on high heat for 18 minutes, or until pasta becomes al dente

Add 1 cup of cheese and stir.

Sprinkle with the remaining vegan cheese and garnishing ingredients

Pappardelle Pasta with Tomatoes and Vegan Cheese

INGREDIENTS

1 red onion, medium chopped

1 green bell pepper chopped

15 ounce can butterbeans, rinsed and drained

15 ounce can black beans , rinsed and drained

28 ounce crushed tomatoes

2 tbsp. tomato paste

1 tsp. basil

1 tsp. Italian seasoning

½ teaspoon salt

1/8 teaspoon black pepper

2 cups vegetable stock

8 ounces pappardelle pasta uncooked

1 ½ cups Vegan Cheese (Tofu Based)

Garnishing ingredients:

chopped green onions for serving

Put all of the ingredients except for pasta, vegan cheese, and garnishing ingredients in your slow cooker.

Combine and cover.

Cook on high heat for 4 hours or low heat for 7 hours.

Add the pasta and cooking on high heat for 18 minutes, or until pasta becomes al dente

Add 1 cup of cheese and stir.

Sprinkle with the remaining vegan cheese and garnishing ingredients

Macaroni and Garbanzo Beans

INGREDIENTS

15 ounce can pinto beans rinsed and drained

15 ounce can garbanzo beans rinsed and drained

28 ounce crushed tomatoes

4 tbsp. pesto

1 tsp. Italian seasoning

½ teaspoon salt

1/8 teaspoon black pepper

2 cups vegetable stock

8 ounces whole wheat elbow macaroni pasta uncooked

1 ½ cups Vegan Cheese (Tofu Based)

Garnishing ingredients:

chopped green onions for serving

Put all of the ingredients except for pasta, vegan cheese, and garnishing ingredients in your slow cooker.

Combine and cover.

Cook on high heat for 4 hours or low heat for 7 hours.

Add the pasta and cooking on high heat for 18 minutes, or until pasta becomes al dente

Add 1 cup of cheese and stir.

Sprinkle with the remaining vegan cheese and garnishing ingredients

Butter head Lettuce and Peanut Thai Salad

Ingredients:

8 ounces vegan cheese

6 to 7 cups butter head lettuce, 3 bundles, trimmed

1/4 cucumber, halved lengthwise, then thinly sliced

3 tablespoons snipped chives

16 cherry tomatoes

1/2 cup peanuts

1/4 white onion, sliced

Salt and pepper, to taste

Dressing

1 small shallot, minced

2 tablespoon distilled white vinegar

1/4 cup sesame seed oil

1 tbsp. Thai chili garlic sauce

Prep

Combine all of the dressing ingredients in a food processor.

Toss with the rest of the ingredients and combine well.

Lettuce Chives and Pistachio Salad

Ingredients:

7 cups loose leaf lettuce, 3 bundles, trimmed

1/4 European or seedless cucumber, halved lengthwise, then thinly sliced

3 tablespoons chopped or snipped chives

16 grapes

1/2 cup pistachios

1/4 onion, sliced

Salt and pepper, to taste

6 ounces vegan cheese

Dressing

1 sprig parsley, chopped

1 tablespoon distilled white vinegar

1/4 lemon, juiced, about 2 teaspoons

1/4 cup extra-virgin olive oil

Prep

Combine all of the dressing ingredients in a food processor.

Toss with the rest of the ingredients and combine well.

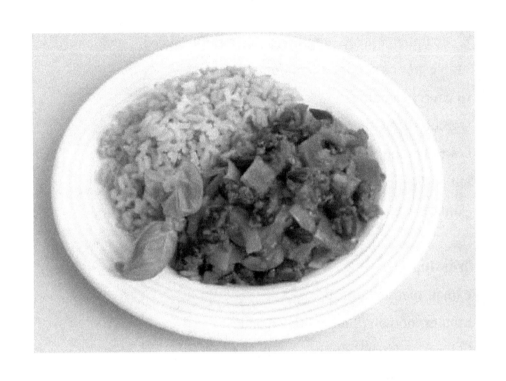

Lettuce Almond and Vegan Cream Cheese Salad

Ingredients:

7 cups frisee lettuce, 3 bundles, trimmed

½ cucumber, halved lengthwise, then thinly sliced

3 tablespoons chopped or snipped chives

16 cherry tomatoes

1/2 cup sliced almonds

1/4 red onion, sliced

Salt and pepper, to taste

7 ounces vegan cream cheese

Dressing

1 small shallot, minced

1 tablespoon distilled white vinegar

1/4 lemon, juiced, about 2 teaspoons

1/4 cup extra-virgin olive oil

1 tbsp. chimichurri sauce

Prep

Combine all of the dressing ingredients in a food processor.

Toss with the rest of the ingredients and combine well.

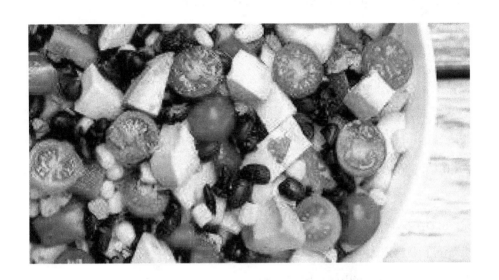

Boston Lettuce and Tomato Salad d

Ingredients:

6 to 7 cups Boston lettuce, 3 bundles, trimmed

1/4 cucumber, halved lengthwise, then thinly sliced

3 tablespoons chopped or snipped chives

16 cherry tomatoes

1/2 cup sliced almonds

1/4 red onion, sliced

Salt and pepper, to taste

5 ounces vegan cheese

Dressing

1 sprig parsley, minced

1 tablespoon distilled white vinegar

1/4 lemon, juiced, about 2 teaspoons

1/4 cup extra-virgin olive oil

Prep

Combine all of the dressing ingredients in a food processor.

Toss with the rest of the ingredients and combine well.

Lettuce and Tomato with Cilantro Vinaigrette

Ingredients:

6 to 7 cups ice berg lettuce, 3 bundles, trimmed

1/4 cucumber, halved lengthwise, then thinly sliced

3 tablespoons chopped or snipped chives

16 cherry tomatoes

1/2 cup sliced almonds

1/4 white onion, sliced

Salt and pepper, to taste

8 ounces vegan cheese

Dressing

1 sprig cilantro, minced

1 tablespoon distilled white vinegar

1/4 lemon, juiced, about 2 teaspoons

1/4 cup extra-virgin olive oil

Prep

Combine all of the dressing ingredients in a food processor.

Toss with the rest of the ingredients and combine well.

Mixed Greens and Almond Salad

Ingredients:

7 cups mesclun, 3 bundles, trimmed

1/4 cucumber, halved lengthwise, then thinly sliced

3 tablespoons chopped or snipped chives

16 cherry tomatoes

1/2 cup sliced almonds

1/4 white onion, sliced

Salt and pepper, to taste

8 ounces vegan cheese

Dressing

1 tablespoon distilled white vinegar

1/4 lemon, juiced, about 2 teaspoons

1/4 cup extra-virgin olive oil

1 tsp. English mustard

Prep

Combine all of the dressing ingredients in a food processor.

Toss with the rest of the ingredients and combine well.

Chervil and Vegan Ricotta Salad

Ingredients:

6 to 7 cups chervil, 3 bundles, trimmed

1/4 cucumber, halved lengthwise, then thinly sliced

16 grapes

1/2 cup sliced almonds

1/4 white onion, sliced

Salt and pepper, to taste

8 ounces Tofu Ricotta Cheese (Tofitti)

Dressing

1 tablespoon distilled white vinegar

1/4 lemon, juiced, about 2 teaspoons

1/4 cup extra-virgin olive oil

1 tbsp. Chimichurri sauce

Prep

Combine all of the dressing ingredients in a food processor.

Toss with the rest of the ingredients and combine well.

Bib Lettuce Walnut and Vegan Parmesan Salad

Ingredients:

6 to 7 cups bib lettuce, 3 bundles, trimmed

1/4 cucumber, halved lengthwise, then thinly sliced

3 tablespoons chopped or snipped chives

16 tomatillos, sliced in half

1/2 cup walnuts

1/4 red onion, sliced

Salt and pepper, to taste

Vegan Parmesan Cheese (Angel Food)

Dressing

1 tablespoon distilled white vinegar

1/4 lemon, juiced, about 2 teaspoons

1/4 cup extra-virgin olive oil

1 tsp. egg free mayonnaise

Prep

Combine all of the dressing ingredients in a food processor.

Toss with the rest of the ingredients and combine well.

Endive Lettuce Tomatillo and Vegan Ricotta Salad

Ingredients:

6 to 7 cups endive lettuce, 3 bundles, trimmed

1/4 cucumber, halved lengthwise, then thinly sliced

3 tablespoons chopped or snipped chives

16 green tomatillos, sliced in half

1/2 cup sliced almonds

1/4 white onion, sliced

Salt and pepper, to taste

8 ounces Tofu Ricotta Cheese (Tofitti)

Dressing

1 tablespoon distilled white vinegar

1/4 lemon, juiced, about 2 teaspoons

1/4 cup extra-virgin olive oil

1 tsp. Dijon mustard

Prep

Combine all of the dressing ingredients in a food processor.

Toss with the rest of the ingredients and combine well.

Kale Tomato and Vegan Parmesan Salad

Ingredients:

6 to 7 cups kale lettuce, 3 bundles, trimmed

1/4 cucumber, halved lengthwise, then thinly sliced

3 tablespoons chopped or snipped chives

16 cherry tomatoes

1/2 cup sliced almonds

1/4 white onion, sliced

Salt and pepper, to taste

Vegan Parmesan Cheese (Angel Food)

Dressing

1 sprig cilantro, minced

1 tablespoon distilled white vinegar

1/4 lemon, juiced, about 2 teaspoons

1/4 cup extra-virgin olive oil

1 tsp. egg free mayonnaise

Prep

Combine all of the dressing ingredients in a food processor.

Toss with the rest of the ingredients and combine well.

Spinach Tomatillos and Almond Salad

Ingredients:

6 to 7 cups spinach lettuce, 3 bundles, trimmed

1/4 cucumber, halved lengthwise, then thinly sliced

3 tablespoons chopped or snipped chives

16 tomatillos, sliced in half

1/2 cup sliced almonds

1/4 white onion, sliced

Salt and pepper, to taste

8 ounces vegan cheese

Dressing

1 sprig cilantro, minced

1 tablespoon distilled white vinegar

1/4 lemon, juiced, about 2 teaspoons

1/4 cup extra-virgin olive oil

1 tsp. English mustard

Prep

Combine all of the dressing ingredients in a food processor.

Toss with the rest of the ingredients and combine well.

Kale Tomato and Almond Salad

Ingredients:

6 to 7 cups kale, 3 bundles, trimmed

1/4 cucumber, halved lengthwise, then thinly sliced

3 tablespoons chopped or snipped chives

16 cherry tomatoes

1/2 cup sliced almonds

1/4 white onion, sliced

Salt and pepper, to taste

8 ounces vegan cheese

Dressing

1 sprig cilantro, minced

1 tablespoon distilled white vinegar

1/4 lemon, juiced, about 2 teaspoons

1/4 cup extra-virgin olive oil

1 tsp. English mustard

Prep

Combine all of the dressing ingredients in a food processor.

Toss with the rest of the ingredients and combine well.

Mixed Green Almond and Vegan Ricotta Salad

Ingredients:

6 to 7 cups mesclun, 3 bundles, trimmed

1/4 cucumber, halved lengthwise, then thinly sliced

3 tablespoons chopped or snipped chives

16 green tomatillos, sliced in half

1/2 cup sliced almonds

1/4 white onion, sliced

Salt and pepper, to taste

8 ounces Tofu Ricotta Cheese (Tofitti)

Dressing

1 tablespoon distilled white vinegar

1/4 lemon, juiced, about 2 teaspoons

1/4 cup extra-virgin olive oil

1 tsp. Dijon mustard

Prep

Combine all of the dressing ingredients in a food processor.

Toss with the rest of the ingredients and combine well.

Endive Tomato and Almond Salad

Ingredients:

6 to 7 cups endive, 3 bundles, trimmed

1/4 cucumber, halved lengthwise, then thinly sliced

3 tablespoons chopped or snipped chives

16 cherry tomatoes

1/2 cup sliced almonds

1/4 white onion, sliced

Salt and pepper, to taste

Vegan Parmesan Cheese (Angel Food)

Dressing

1 sprig cilantro, minced

1 tablespoon distilled white vinegar

1/4 lemon, juiced, about 2 teaspoons

1/4 cup extra-virgin olive oil

1 tsp. English mustard

Prep

Combine all of the dressing ingredients in a food processor.

Toss with the rest of the ingredients and combine well.

Kale Tomatillo and Almond Salad

Ingredients:

6 to 7 cups kale, 3 bundles, trimmed

1/4 cucumber, halved lengthwise, then thinly sliced

3 tablespoons chopped or snipped chives

16 tomatillos, sliced in half

1/2 cup sliced almonds

1/4 white onion, sliced

Salt and pepper, to taste

8 ounces Tofu Ricotta Cheese (Tofitti)

Dressing

1 tablespoon distilled white vinegar

1/4 lemon, juiced, about 2 teaspoons

1/4 cup extra-virgin olive oil

1 tsp. egg-free mayonnaise

Prep

Combine all of the dressing ingredients in a food processor.

Toss with the rest of the ingredients and combine well.

Escarole Almond and Tomato Salad

Ingredients:

6 to 7 cups escarole, 3 bundles, trimmed

1/4 cucumber, halved lengthwise, then thinly sliced

3 tablespoons chopped or snipped chives

16 cherry tomatoes

1/2 cup sliced almonds

1/4 white onion, sliced

Salt and pepper, to taste

8 ounces vegan cheese

Dressing

1 sprig cilantro, minced

1 tablespoon distilled white vinegar

1/4 lemon, juiced, about 2 teaspoons

1/4 cup extra-virgin olive oil

1 tsp. English mustard

Prep

Combine all of the dressing ingredients in a food processor.

Toss with the rest of the ingredients and combine well.

Endive Tomatillo and Almond Salad

Ingredients:

6 to 7 cups endive, 3 bundles, trimmed

1/4 cucumber, halved lengthwise, then thinly sliced

3 tablespoons chopped or snipped chives

16 tomatillos, sliced in half

1/2 cup sliced almonds

1/4 white onion, sliced

Salt and pepper, to taste

Vegan Parmesan Cheese (Angel Food)

Dressing

1 tablespoon distilled white vinegar

1/4 lemon, juiced, about 2 teaspoons

1/4 cup extra-virgin olive oil

1 tsp. Dijon mustard

Prep

Combine all of the dressing ingredients in a food processor.

Toss with the rest of the ingredients and combine well.

Bib Lettuce Almond and Cherry Tomato Salad

Ingredients:

6 to 7 cups bib lettuce, 3 bundles, trimmed

1/4 cucumber, halved lengthwise, then thinly sliced

3 tablespoons chopped or snipped chives

16 cherry tomatoes

1/2 cup sliced almonds

1/4 white onion, sliced

Salt and pepper, to taste

8 ounces Tofu Ricotta Cheese (Tofitti)

Dressing

1 sprig cilantro, minced

1 tablespoon distilled white vinegar

1/4 lemon, juiced, about 2 teaspoons

1/4 cup extra-virgin olive oil

1 tsp. English mustard

Prep

Combine all of the dressing ingredients in a food processor.

Toss with the rest of the ingredients and combine well.

Spinach Tomatillos and Vegan Parmesan Salad

Ingredients:

6 to 7 cups spinach lettuce, 3 bundles, trimmed

1/4 cucumber, halved lengthwise, then thinly sliced

3 tablespoons chopped or snipped chives

16 tomatillos, sliced in half

1/2 cup sliced almonds

1/4 white onion, sliced

Salt and pepper, to taste

Vegan Parmesan Cheese (Angel Food)

Dressing

1 sprig cilantro, minced

1 tablespoon distilled white vinegar

1/4 lemon, juiced, about 2 teaspoons

1/4 cup extra-virgin olive oil

1 tsp. egg free mayonnaise

Prep

Combine all of the dressing ingredients in a food processor.

Toss with the rest of the ingredients and combine well.

Kale Tomato and Vegan Parmesan Cheese Salad

Ingredients:

6 to 7 cups kale lettuce, 3 bundles, trimmed

1/4 cucumber, halved lengthwise, then thinly sliced

3 tablespoons chopped or snipped chives

16 cherry tomatoes

1/2 cup sliced almonds

1/4 white onion, sliced

Salt and pepper, to taste

Vegan Parmesan Cheese (Angel Food)

Dressing

1 sprig cilantro, minced

1 tablespoon distilled white vinegar

1/4 lemon, juiced, about 2 teaspoons

1/4 cup extra-virgin olive oil

1 tsp. English mustard

Prep

Combine all of the dressing ingredients in a food processor.

Toss with the rest of the ingredients and combine well.

Mixed Greens Tomatillo and Vegan Ricotta Cheese Salad

Ingredients:

6 to 7 cups mesclun, 3 bundles, trimmed

1/4 cucumber, halved lengthwise, then thinly sliced

3 tablespoons chopped or snipped chives

16 green tomatillos, sliced in half

1/2 cup sliced almonds

1/4 white onion, sliced

Salt and pepper, to taste

8 ounces Tofu Ricotta Cheese (Tofitti)

Dressing

1 sprig cilantro, minced

1 tablespoon distilled white vinegar

1/4 lemon, juiced, about 2 teaspoons

1/4 cup extra-virgin olive oil

Prep

Combine all of the dressing ingredients in a food processor.

Toss with the rest of the ingredients and combine well.

Escarole Almond and Vegan Ricotta Cheese Salad

Ingredients:

6 to 7 cups escarole, 3 bundles, trimmed

1/4 cucumber, halved lengthwise, then thinly sliced

3 tablespoons chopped or snipped chives

16 tomatillos, sliced in half

1/2 cup sliced almonds

1/4 white onion, sliced

Salt and pepper, to taste

8 ounces Tofu Ricotta Cheese (Tofitti)

Dressing

1 tablespoon distilled white vinegar

1/4 lemon, juiced, about 2 teaspoons

1/4 cup extra-virgin olive oil

1 tsp. Dijon mustard

Prep

Combine all of the dressing ingredients in a food processor.

Toss with the rest of the ingredients and combine well.

Endive Tomato and Almond Salad

Ingredients:

6 to 7 cups endive, 3 bundles, trimmed

1/4 cucumber, halved lengthwise, then thinly sliced

3 tablespoons chopped or snipped chives

16 cherry tomatoes

1/2 cup sliced almonds

1/4 white onion, sliced

Salt and pepper, to taste

8 ounces vegan cheese

Dressing

1 sprig cilantro, minced

1 tablespoon distilled white vinegar

1/4 lemon, juiced, about 2 teaspoons

1/4 cup extra-virgin olive oil

1 tsp. egg free mayonnaise

Prep

Combine all of the dressing ingredients in a food processor.

Toss with the rest of the ingredients and combine well.

Spinach Zucchini and Almond Salad

Ingredients:

6 to 7 cups spinach, 3 bundles, trimmed

¼ zucchini, halved lengthwise, then thinly sliced

3 tablespoons chopped or snipped chives

16 cherry tomatoes

1/2 cup sliced almonds

1/4 white onion, sliced

Salt and pepper, to taste

8 ounces vegan cheese

Dressing

1 tablespoon distilled white vinegar

1/4 lemon, juiced, about 2 teaspoons

1/4 cup extra-virgin olive oil

1 tsp. pesto sauce

Prep

Combine all of the dressing ingredients in a food processor.

Toss with the rest of the ingredients and combine well.

Kale Cucumber Tomatillo and Tofu Ricotta Salad

Ingredients:

6 to 7 cups kale, 3 bundles, trimmed

1/4 cucumber, halved lengthwise, then thinly sliced

3 tablespoons chopped or snipped chives

16 green tomatillos, sliced in half

1/2 cup sliced almonds

1/4 white onion, sliced

Salt and pepper, to taste

8 ounces Tofu Ricotta Cheese (Tofitti)

Dressing

1 sprig cilantro, minced

1 tablespoon distilled white vinegar

1/4 lemon, juiced, about 2 teaspoons

1/4 cup extra-virgin olive oil

1 tsp. English mustard

Prep

Combine all of the dressing ingredients in a food processor.

Toss with the rest of the ingredients and combine well.

Mixed Greens Almond and Tofu Ricotta Salad

Ingredients:

6 to 7 cups mesclun, 3 bundles, trimmed

1/4 cucumber, halved lengthwise, then thinly sliced

3 tablespoons chopped or snipped chives

16 tomatillos, sliced in half

1/2 cup sliced almonds

1/4 white onion, sliced

Salt and pepper, to taste

8 ounces Tofu Ricotta Cheese (Tofitti)

Dressing

1 sprig cilantro, minced

1 tablespoon distilled white vinegar

1/4 lemon, juiced, about 2 teaspoons

1/4 cup extra-virgin olive oil

1 tsp. egg free mayonnaise

Prep

Combine all of the dressing ingredients in a food processor.

Toss with the rest of the ingredients and combine well.

Kale Tomato and Vegan Parmesan Cheese Salad

Ingredients:

6 to 7 cups kale, 3 bundles, trimmed

1/4 cucumber, halved lengthwise, then thinly sliced

3 tablespoons chopped or snipped chives

16 cherry tomatoes

1/2 cup sliced almonds

1/4 white onion, sliced

Salt and pepper, to taste

Vegan Parmesan Cheese (Angel Food)

Dressing

1 sprig cilantro, minced

1 tablespoon distilled white vinegar

1/4 lemon, juiced, about 2 teaspoons

1/4 cup extra-virgin olive oil

1 tsp. English mustard

Prep

Combine all of the dressing ingredients in a food processor.

Toss with the rest of the ingredients and combine well.

Chervil Tomato and Vegan Parmesan Cheese Salad

Ingredients:

6 to 7 cups chervil, 3 bundles, trimmed

1/4 cucumber, halved lengthwise, then thinly sliced

3 tablespoons chopped or snipped chives

16 cherry tomatoes

1/2 cup sliced almonds

1/4 white onion, sliced

Salt and pepper, to taste

Vegan Parmesan Cheese (Angel Food)

Dressing

1 sprig cilantro, minced

1 tablespoon distilled white vinegar

1/4 lemon, juiced, about 2 teaspoons

1/4 cup extra-virgin olive oil

1 tsp. English mustard

Prep

Combine all of the dressing ingredients in a food processor.

Toss with the rest of the ingredients and combine well.

Bib Lettuce Tomatillo and Tofu Ricotta Cheese Salad

Ingredients:

6 to 7 cups bib lettuce, 3 bundles, trimmed

1/4 cucumber, halved lengthwise, then thinly sliced

3 tablespoons chopped or snipped chives

16 green tomatillos, sliced in half

1/2 cup sliced almonds

1/4 white onion, sliced

Salt and pepper, to taste

8 ounces Tofu Ricotta Cheese (Tofitti)

Dressing

1 sprig cilantro, minced

1 tablespoon distilled white vinegar

1/4 lemon, juiced, about 2 teaspoons

1/4 cup extra-virgin olive oil

1 tsp. egg free mayonnaise

Prep

Combine all of the dressing ingredients in a food processor.

Toss with the rest of the ingredients and combine well.

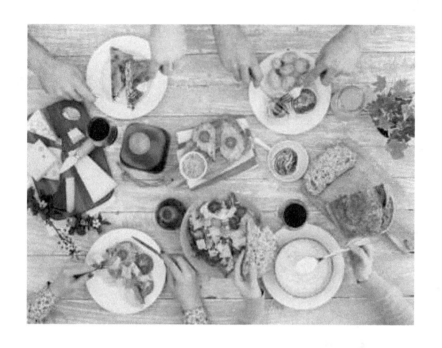

Spinach Tomatoes & Almond Salad

Ingredients:

6 to 7 cups spinach, 3 bundles, trimmed

1/4 cucumber, halved lengthwise, then thinly sliced

3 tablespoons chopped or snipped chives

16 cherry tomatoes

1/2 cup sliced almonds

1/4 white onion, sliced

Salt and pepper, to taste

8 ounces vegan cheese

Dressing

1 sprig cilantro, minced

1 tablespoon distilled white vinegar

1/4 lemon, juiced, about 2 teaspoons

1/4 cup extra-virgin olive oil

1 tsp. English mustard

Prep

Combine all of the dressing ingredients in a food processor.

Toss with the rest of the ingredients and combine well.

Napa Cabbage Tomatillo and Vegan Parmesan Cheese Salad

Ingredients:

6 to 7 cups Napa cabbage, 3 bundles, trimmed

1/4 cucumber, halved lengthwise, then thinly sliced

3 tablespoons chopped or snipped chives

16 tomatillos, sliced in half

1/2 cup sliced almonds

1/4 white onion, sliced

Salt and pepper, to taste

Vegan Parmesan Cheese (Angel Food)

Dressing

1 sprig cilantro, minced

1 tablespoon distilled white vinegar

1/4 lemon, juiced, about 2 teaspoons

1/4 cup extra-virgin olive oil

Prep

Combine all of the dressing ingredients in a food processor.

Toss with the rest of the ingredients and combine well.

Chicory Tomatillo and Almond Salad

Ingredients:

6 to 7 cups chicory, 3 bundles, trimmed

1/4 cucumber, halved lengthwise, then thinly sliced

3 tablespoons chopped or snipped chives

16 green tomatillos, sliced in half

1/2 cup sliced almonds

1/4 white onion, sliced

Salt and pepper, to taste

Vegan Parmesan Cheese (Angel Food)

Dressing

1 sprig cilantro, minced

1 tablespoon distilled white vinegar

1/4 lemon, juiced, about 2 teaspoons

1/4 cup extra-virgin olive oil

1 tsp. English mustard

Prep

Combine all of the dressing ingredients in a food processor.

Toss with the rest of the ingredients and combine well.

Kale Tomatoes and Tofu Ricotta Cheese Salad

Ingredients:

6 to 7 cups kale, 3 bundles, trimmed

1/4 cucumber, halved lengthwise, then thinly sliced

3 tablespoons chopped or snipped chives

16 cherry tomatoes

1/2 cup sliced almonds

1/4 white onion, sliced

Salt and pepper, to taste

8 ounces Tofu Ricotta Cheese (Tofitti)

Dressing

1 sprig cilantro, minced

1 tablespoon distilled white vinegar

1/4 lemon, juiced, about 2 teaspoons

1/4 cup extra-virgin olive oil

1 tsp. egg free mayonnaise

Prep

Combine all of the dressing ingredients in a food processor.

Toss with the rest of the ingredients and combine well.

Napa Cabbage Tomatoes and Tofu ricotta Cheese Salad

Ingredients:

6 to 7 cups Napa cabbage, 3 bundles, trimmed

1/4 cucumber, halved lengthwise, then thinly sliced

3 tablespoons chopped or snipped chives

16 cherry tomatoes

1/2 cup sliced almonds

1/4 white onion, sliced

Salt and pepper, to taste

8 ounces Tofu Ricotta Cheese (Tofitti)

Dressing

1 sprig cilantro, minced

1 tablespoon distilled white vinegar

1/4 lemon, juiced, about 2 teaspoons

1/4 cup extra-virgin olive oil

Prep

Combine all of the dressing ingredients in a food processor.

Toss with the rest of the ingredients and combine well.

Baby Beet Greens Tomatillos and Vegan Cheese Salad

Ingredients:

6 to 7 cups baby beet greens, 3 bundles, trimmed

1/4 cucumber, halved lengthwise, then thinly sliced

3 tablespoons chopped or snipped chives

16 tomatillos, sliced in half

1/2 cup sliced almonds

1/4 white onion, sliced

Salt and pepper, to taste

8 ounces vegan cheese

Dressing

1 sprig cilantro, minced

1 tablespoon distilled white vinegar

1/4 lemon, juiced, about 2 teaspoons

1/4 cup extra-virgin olive oil

1 tsp. English mustard

Prep

Combine all of the dressing ingredients in a food processor.

Toss with the rest of the ingredients and combine well.

Super Simple Romaine Lettuce Salad

Ingredients:

1 head romaine lettuce, rinsed, patted and shredded

Dressing

1/2 cup white wine vinegar

1 tablespoon extra virgin olive oil

Freshly ground black pepper

3/4 cup finely ground almonds

Sea salt

Prep

Combine all of the dressing ingredients in a food processor.

Toss with the rest of the ingredients and combine well.

Easy Bib Lettuce Salad

Ingredients:

1 head bib lettuce, rinsed, patted and shredded

Dressing

2 tbsp. white wine vinegar

4 tablespoons macadamia oil

Freshly ground black pepper

3/4 cup finely ground peanuts

Sea salt

Prep

Combine all of the dressing ingredients in a food processor.

Toss with the rest of the ingredients and combine well.

Easy Boston Salad

Ingredients:

1 head Boston lettuce, rinsed, patted and shredded

Dressing

2 tbsp. apple cider vinegar

4 tablespoons olive oil

Freshly ground black pepper

3/4 cup finely coarsely ground walnuts

Sea salt

Prep

Combine all of the dressing ingredients in a food processor.

Toss with the rest of the ingredients and combine well.

Easy Mixed Greens Salad

Ingredients:

Handful of Mesclun, rinsed, patted and shredded

Dressing

2 tbsp. apple cider vinegar

4 tablespoons olive oil

Freshly ground black pepper

3/4 cup finely coarsely ground hazelnuts

Sea salt

Prep

Combine all of the dressing ingredients in a food processor.

Toss with the rest of the ingredients and combine well.

Bib Lettuce Salad

Ingredients:

1 head bib lettuce, rinsed, patted and shredded

Dressing

2 tbsp. balsamic vinegar

4 tablespoons extra virgin olive oil

Freshly ground black pepper

3/4 cup finely ground peanuts

Sea salt

Prep

Combine all of the dressing ingredients in a food processor.

Toss with the rest of the ingredients and combine well.

Boston Lettuce Salad with Balsamic Glaze

Ingredients:

1 head Boston lettuce, rinsed, patted and shredded

Dressing

2 tbsp. balsamic vinegar

4 tablespoons macadamia oil

Freshly ground black pepper

3/4 cup finely ground almonds

Sea salt

Prep

Combine all of the dressing ingredients in a food processor.

Toss with the rest of the ingredients and combine well.

Simple Endive Salad

Ingredients:

1 Head of Endive, rinsed, patted and shredded

Dressing

2 tbsp. white wine vinegar

4 tablespoons extra virgin olive oil

Freshly ground black pepper

3/4 cup finely coarsely ground walnuts

Sea salt

Prep

Combine all of the dressing ingredients in a food processor.

Toss with the rest of the ingredients and combine well.

Mixed Greens Salad

Ingredients:

Handful of Mesclun, rinsed, patted and shredded

Dressing

2 tbsp. distilled white vinegar

4 tablespoons extra virgin olive oil

Freshly ground black pepper

3/4 cup finely coarsely ground cashews

Sea salt

Prep

Combine all of the dressing ingredients in a food processor.

Toss with the rest of the ingredients and combine well.

Boston Lettuce and Peanut Salad

Ingredients:

1 head Boston lettuce, rinsed, patted and shredded

Dressing

2 tbsp. apple cider vinegar

4 tablespoons olive oil

Freshly ground black pepper

3/4 cup finely ground peanuts

Sea salt

Prep

Combine all of the dressing ingredients in a food processor.

Toss with the rest of the ingredients and combine well.

Boston Lettuce with Balsamic Glaze

Ingredients:

1 head Boston lettuce, rinsed, patted and shredded

Dressing

2 tbsp. balsamic vinegar

4 tablespoons macadamia oil

Freshly ground black pepper

3/4 cup finely coarsely ground hazelnuts

Sea salt

Prep

Combine all of the dressing ingredients in a food processor.

Toss with the rest of the ingredients and combine well.

Bib Lettuce with Walnut Vinaigrette

Ingredients:

1 head bib lettuce, rinsed, patted and shredded

Dressing

2 tbsp. distilled white vinegar

4 tablespoons extra virgin olive oil

Freshly ground black pepper

3/4 cup finely coarsely ground walnuts

Sea salt

Prep

Combine all of the dressing ingredients in a food processor.

Toss with the rest of the ingredients and combine well.

Romaine Lettuce with Hazelnut Vinaigrette

Ingredients:

1 head romaine lettuce, rinsed, patted and shredded

Dressing

2 tbsp. apple cider vinegar

4 tablespoons extra virgin olive oil

Freshly ground black pepper

3/4 cup finely coarsely ground hazelnuts

Sea salt

Prep

Combine all of the dressing ingredients in a food processor.

Toss with the rest of the ingredients and combine well.

Mixed Greens with Almond Vinaigrette Salad

Ingredients:

Handful of Mesclun, rinsed, patted and shredded

Dressing

2 tbsp. white wine vinegar

4 tablespoons olive oil

Freshly ground black pepper

3/4 cup finely ground almonds

Sea salt

Prep

Combine all of the dressing ingredients in a food processor.

Toss with the rest of the ingredients and combine well.

Endive with Peanut and Balsamic Vinaigrette Salad

Ingredients:

1 Head of Endive, rinsed, patted and shredded

Dressing

2 tbsp. balsamic vinegar

4 tablespoons extra virgin olive oil

Freshly ground black pepper

3/4 cup finely ground peanuts

Sea salt

Prep

Combine all of the dressing ingredients in a food processor.

Toss with the rest of the ingredients and combine well.

Bib Lettuce with Cashew Vinaigrette

Ingredients:

1 head bib lettuce, rinsed, patted and shredded

Dressing

2 tbsp. distilled white vinegar

4 tablespoons macadamia oil

Freshly ground black pepper

3/4 cup finely coarsely ground cashews

Sea salt

Prep

Combine all of the dressing ingredients in a food processor.

Toss with the rest of the ingredients and combine well.

Romaine Lettuce with Walnut Vinaigrette Salad

Ingredients:

1 head romaine lettuce, rinsed, patted and shredded

Dressing

2 tbsp. red wine vinegar

1 tablespoon extra virgin olive oil

Freshly ground black pepper

3/4 cup finely coarsely ground walnuts

Sea salt

Prep

Combine all of the dressing ingredients in a food processor.

Toss with the rest of the ingredients and combine well.

Mixed Greens with Almond Vinaigrette Salad

Ingredients:

Handful of Mesclun, rinsed, patted and shredded

Dressing

2 tbsp. balsamic vinegar

1 tablespoon extra virgin olive oil

Freshly ground black pepper

3/4 cup finely ground almonds

Sea salt

Prep

Combine all of the dressing ingredients in a food processor.

Toss with the rest of the ingredients and combine well.

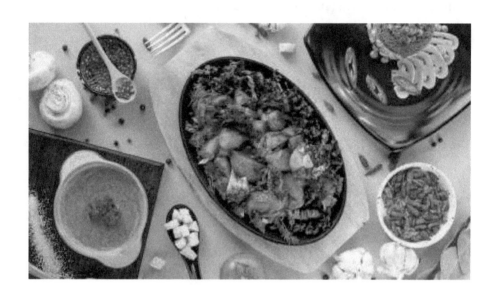

Romaine Lettuce with Cashew Vinaigrette Salad

Ingredients:

1 head romaine lettuce, rinsed, patted and shredded

Dressing

2 tbsp. apple cider vinegar

4 tablespoons olive oil

Freshly ground black pepper

3/4 cup finely coarsely ground cashews

Sea salt

Prep

Combine all of the dressing ingredients in a food processor.

Toss with the rest of the ingredients and combine well.

Endive with Hazelnut Vinaigrette Salad

Ingredients:

1 Head of Endive, rinsed, patted and shredded

Dressing

2 tbsp. white wine vinegar

4 tablespoons extra virgin olive oil

Freshly ground black pepper

3/4 cup finely coarsely ground hazelnuts

Sea salt

Prep

Combine all of the dressing ingredients in a food processor.

Toss with the rest of the ingredients and combine well.

Bib Lettuce with Peanut Vinaigrette Salad

Ingredients:

1 head bib lettuce, rinsed, patted and shredded

Dressing

2 tbsp. distilled white vinegar

4 tablespoons macadamia oil

Freshly ground black pepper

3/4 cup finely ground peanuts

Sea salt

Prep

Combine all of the dressing ingredients in a food processor.

Toss with the rest of the ingredients and combine well.

Grilles Boston Lettuce Salad

Ingredients:

1 head Boston lettuce, rinsed, patted and shredded

Dressing

2 tbsp. white wine vinegar

4 tablespoons extra virgin olive oil

Freshly ground black pepper

3/4 cup finely ground almonds

Sea salt

Prep

Grill the lettuce and/or greens over medium heat until lightly charred

Combine all of the dressing ingredients in a food processor.

Toss with the rest of the ingredients and combine well.

Grilled Romaine Lettuce Salad

Ingredients:

1 head romaine lettuce, rinsed, patted and shredded

Dressing

2 tbsp. balsamic vinegar

4 tablespoons extra virgin olive oil

Freshly ground black pepper

3/4 cup finely ground peanuts

Sea salt

Prep

Grill the lettuce and/or greens over medium heat until lightly charred

Combine all of the dressing ingredients in a food processor.

Toss with the rest of the ingredients and combine well.

Grilled Romaine Lettuce and Cashew Vinaigrette Salad

Ingredients:

1 head romaine lettuce, rinsed, patted and shredded

Dressing

2 tbsp. red wine vinegar

4 tablespoons olive oil

Freshly ground black pepper

3/4 cup finely coarsely ground cashews

Sea salt

Prep

Grill the lettuce and/or greens over medium heat until lightly charred

Combine all of the dressing ingredients in a food processor.

Toss with the rest of the ingredients and combine well.

Grilled Romaine Lettuce and Almond Vinaigrette Salad

Ingredients:

1 head romaine lettuce, rinsed, patted and shredded

Dressing

2 tbsp. red wine vinegar

4 tablespoons extra virgin olive oil

Freshly ground black pepper

3/4 cup finely ground almonds

Sea salt

Prep

Grill the lettuce and/or greens over medium heat until lightly charred

Combine all of the dressing ingredients in a food processor.

Toss with the rest of the ingredients and combine well.

Grilled Napa Cabbage with Cashew Vinaigrette

Ingredients:

1 head Napa cabbage, rinsed, patted and shredded

½ cup capers

Dressing

2 tbsp. balsamic vinegar

4 tablespoons macadamia oil

Freshly ground black pepper

3/4 cup finely coarsely ground cashews

Sea salt

Prep

Grill the lettuce and/or greens over medium heat until lightly charred

Combine all of the dressing ingredients in a food processor.

Toss with the rest of the ingredients and combine well.

Grilled Boston lettuce and Cashew Vinaigrette Salad

Ingredients:

1 head Boston lettuce, rinsed, patted and shredded

½ cup green olives

Dressing

2 tbsp. white wine vinegar

4 tablespoons extra virgin olive oil

Freshly ground black pepper

3/4 cup finely coarsely ground cashews

Sea salt

Prep

Grill the lettuce and/or greens over medium heat until lightly charred

Combine all of the dressing ingredients in a food processor.

Toss with the rest of the ingredients and combine well.

Grilled Romaine Lettuce and Green Olives Salad

Ingredients:

1 head romaine lettuce, rinsed, patted and shredded

½ cup green olives

Dressing

2 tbsp. apple cider vinegar

4 tablespoons olive oil

Freshly ground black pepper

3/4 cup finely coarsely ground walnuts

Sea salt

Prep

Grill the lettuce and/or greens over medium heat until lightly charred

Combine all of the dressing ingredients in a food processor.

Toss with the rest of the ingredients and combine well.

Grilled Bib Lettuce and Green Olives Salad

Ingredients:

1 head bib lettuce, rinsed, patted and shredded

½ cup green olives

Dressing

2 tbsp. red wine vinegar

4 tablespoons extra virgin olive oil

Freshly ground black pepper

3/4 cup finely ground almonds

Sea salt

Prep

Grill the lettuce and/or greens over medium heat until lightly charred

Combine all of the dressing ingredients in a food processor.

Toss with the rest of the ingredients and combine well.

Grilled Romaine Lettuce and Green Capers Salad

Ingredients:

1 head romaine lettuce, rinsed, patted and shredded

½ cup green capers

Dressing

2 tbsp. apple cider vinegar

4 tablespoons extra virgin olive oil

Freshly ground black pepper

3/4 cup finely ground peanuts

Sea salt

Prep

Grill the lettuce and/or greens over medium heat until lightly charred

Combine all of the dressing ingredients in a food processor.

Toss with the rest of the ingredients and combine well.

Grilled Romaine Lettuce and Capers Salad

Ingredients:

1 head romaine lettuce, rinsed, patted and shredded

½ cup green capers

Dressing

2 tbsp. white wine vinegar

4 tablespoons extra virgin olive oil

Freshly ground black pepper

3/4 cup finely coarsely ground walnuts

Sea salt

Prep

Grill the lettuce and/or greens over medium heat until lightly charred

Combine all of the dressing ingredients in a food processor.

Toss with the rest of the ingredients and combine well.

Grilled Boston and Black Olives Salad

Ingredients:

1 head Boston lettuce, rinsed, patted and shredded

½ cup black olives

Dressing

2 tbsp. balsamic vinegar

4 tablespoons macadamia oil

Freshly ground black pepper

3/4 cup finely coarsely ground cashews

Sea salt

Prep

Grill the lettuce and/or greens over medium heat until lightly charred

Combine all of the dressing ingredients in a food processor.

Toss with the rest of the ingredients and combine well.

Grilled Romaine Lettuce and Kalamata Olives Salad

Ingredients:

1 head romaine lettuce, rinsed, patted and shredded

½ cup Kalamata olives

Dressing

2 tbsp. red wine vinegar

4 tablespoons olive oil

Freshly ground black pepper

3/4 cup finely ground almonds

Sea salt

Prep

Grill the lettuce and/or greens over medium heat until lightly charred

Combine all of the dressing ingredients in a food processor.

Toss with the rest of the ingredients and combine well.

Romaine Lettuce with Green Olives and Peanut Vinaigrette

Ingredients:

1 head romaine lettuce, rinsed, patted and shredded

½ cup green olives

Dressing

2 tbsp. apple cider vinegar

4 tablespoons extra virgin olive oil

Freshly ground black pepper

3/4 cup finely ground peanuts

Sea salt

Prep

Combine all of the dressing ingredients in a food processor.

Toss with the rest of the ingredients and combine well.

Romaine Lettuce Capers and Almond Vinaigrette

Ingredients:

1 head romaine lettuce, rinsed, patted and shredded

½ cup capers

Dressing

2 tbsp. apple cider vinegar

4 tablespoons extra virgin olive oil

Freshly ground black pepper

3/4 cup finely ground almonds

Sea salt

Prep

Combine all of the dressing ingredients in a food processor.

Toss with the rest of the ingredients and combine well.

Boston Lettuce With Artichoke Hearts and Cashew Vinaigrette

Ingredients:

1 head Boston lettuce, rinsed, patted and shredded

½ cup artichoke hearts

Dressing

2 tbsp. white wine vinegar

4 tablespoons extra virgin olive oil

Freshly ground black pepper

3/4 cup finely coarsely ground cashews

Sea salt

Prep

Combine all of the dressing ingredients in a food processor.

Toss with the rest of the ingredients and combine well.

Artichoke and Artichoke Hearts with Balsamic Glaze

Ingredients:

1 artichoke, rinsed &patted

½ cup artichoke hearts

Dressing

2 tbsp. balsamic vinegar

4 tablespoons macadamia oil

Freshly ground black pepper

3/4 cup finely ground peanuts

Sea salt

Prep

Combine all of the dressing ingredients in a food processor.

Toss with the rest of the ingredients and combine well.

Artichoke and Green Olives with Walnut Vinaigrette

Ingredients:

1 artichoke, rinsed & patted

½ cup green olives

Dressing

2 tbsp. red wine vinegar

4 tablespoons extra virgin olive oil

Freshly ground black pepper

3/4 cup finely coarsely ground walnuts

Sea salt

Prep

Combine all of the dressing ingredients in a food processor.

Toss with the rest of the ingredients and combine well.

Romaine Lettuce with Black Olives and Artichoke Hearts

Ingredients:

1 head romaine lettuce, rinsed, patted and shredded

½ cup black olives

½ cup artichoke hearts

Dressing

2 tbsp. apple cider vinegar

4 tablespoons olive oil

Freshly ground black pepper

3/4 cup finely ground almonds

Sea salt

Prep

Combine all of the dressing ingredients in a food processor.

Toss with the rest of the ingredients and combine well.

Artichoke Hearts with Black Olive Salad

Ingredients:

1 head romaine lettuce, rinsed, patted and shredded

½ cup black olives

½ cup artichoke hearts

Dressing

2 tbsp. white wine vinegar

4 tablespoons extra virgin olive oil

Freshly ground black pepper

3/4 cup finely ground peanuts

Sea salt

Prep

Combine all of the dressing ingredients in a food processor.

Toss with the rest of the ingredients and combine well.

Boston Lettuce Black Olive and Artichoke Heart Salad

Ingredients:

1 head Boston lettuce, rinsed, patted and shredded

½ cup black olives

½ cup artichoke hearts

Dressing

2 tbsp. red wine vinegar

4 tablespoons extra virgin olive oil

Freshly ground black pepper

3/4 cup finely ground almonds

Sea salt

Prep

Combine all of the dressing ingredients in a food processor.

Toss with the rest of the ingredients and combine well.

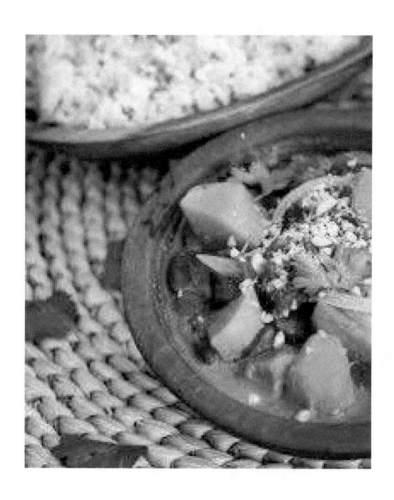

Romaine Lettuce with Artichoke Heart with Macadamia Vinaigrette Salad

Ingredients:

1 head romaine lettuce, rinsed, patted and shredded

½ cup black olives

½ cup artichoke hearts

Dressing

2 tbsp. balsamic vinegar

4 tablespoons macadamia oil

Freshly ground black pepper

3/4 cup finely coarsely ground cashews

Sea salt

Prep

Combine all of the dressing ingredients in a food processor.

Toss with the rest of the ingredients and combine well.

Bib Lettuce Black Olives and Artichoke Heart Salad

Ingredients:

1 head bib lettuce, rinsed, patted and shredded

½ cup black olives

½ cup artichoke hearts

Dressing

2 tbsp. white wine vinegar

4 tablespoons extra virgin olive oil

Freshly ground black pepper

3/4 cup finely ground almonds

Sea salt

Prep

Combine all of the dressing ingredients in a food processor.

Toss with the rest of the ingredients and combine well.

Boston Lettuce with Apple Cider Vinaigrette

Ingredients:

1 head Boston lettuce, rinsed, patted and shredded

½ cup black olives

½ cup artichoke hearts

Dressing

2 tbsp. apple cider vinegar

4 tablespoons extra virgin olive oil

Freshly ground black pepper

3/4 cup finely ground peanuts

Sea salt

Prep

Combine all of the dressing ingredients in a food processor.

Toss with the rest of the ingredients and combine well.

Romaine Lettuce with Artichoke Heart and Cashew Vinaigrette Salad

Ingredients:

1 head romaine lettuce, rinsed, patted and shredded

½ cup black olives

½ cup artichoke hearts

Dressing

2 tbsp. red wine vinegar

4 tablespoons olive oil

Freshly ground black pepper

3/4 cup finely coarsely ground cashews

Sea salt

Prep

Combine all of the dressing ingredients in a food processor.

Toss with the rest of the ingredients and combine well.

Romaine Lettuce Artichoke Heart and Green Olive Salad

Ingredients:

1 head romaine lettuce, rinsed, patted and shredded

½ cup green olives

½ cup artichoke hearts

Dressing

2 tbsp. red wine vinegar

4 tablespoons macadamia oil

Freshly ground black pepper

3/4 cup finely coarsely ground walnuts

Sea salt

Prep

Combine all of the dressing ingredients in a food processor.

Toss with the rest of the ingredients and combine well.

Bib Lettuce Kalamata Olives and Artichoke Heart Salad

Ingredients:

1 head bib lettuce, rinsed, patted and shredded

½ cup Kalamata olives

½ cup artichoke hearts

Dressing

2 tbsp. white wine vinegar

4 tablespoons extra virgin olive oil

Freshly ground black pepper

3/4 cup finely ground almonds

Sea salt

Prep

Combine all of the dressing ingredients in a food processor.

Toss with the rest of the ingredients and combine well.

Romaine Lettuce Baby Corn and Artichoke Heart Salad

Ingredients:

1 head romaine lettuce, rinsed, patted and shredded

½ cup baby corn

½ cup artichoke hearts

Dressing

2 tbsp. balsamic vinegar

4 tablespoons macadamia oil

Freshly ground black pepper

3/4 cup finely coarsely ground cashews

Sea salt

Prep

Combine all of the dressing ingredients in a food processor.

Toss with the rest of the ingredients and combine well.

Boston Lettuce Baby Carrots and Artichoke Heart Salad

Ingredients:

1 head Boston lettuce, rinsed, patted and shredded

½ cup baby carrots

½ cup artichoke hearts

Dressing

2 tbsp. white wine vinegar

4 tablespoons extra virgin olive oil

Freshly ground black pepper

3/4 cup finely ground peanuts

Sea salt

Prep

Combine all of the dressing ingredients in a food processor.

Toss with the rest of the ingredients and combine well.

Romaine Lettuce Black Olives and Baby Corn Salad

Ingredients:

1 head romaine lettuce, rinsed, patted and shredded

½ cup black olives

½ cup canned baby corn

Dressing

2 tbsp. apple cider vinegar

4 tablespoons olive oil

Freshly ground black pepper

3/4 cup finely ground almonds

Sea salt

Prep

Combine all of the dressing ingredients in a food processor.

Toss with the rest of the ingredients and combine well.

Romaine Lettuce & Baby Carrots with Walnut Vinaigrette Salad

Ingredients:

1 head romaine lettuce, rinsed, patted and shredded

½ cup black olives

½ cup baby carrots

Dressing

2 tbsp. white wine vinegar

4 tablespoons extra virgin olive oil

Freshly ground black pepper

3/4 cup finely coarsely ground walnuts

Sea salt

Prep

Combine all of the dressing ingredients in a food processor.

Toss with the rest of the ingredients and combine well.

Boston Lettuce with Capers and Artichoke Heart Salad

Ingredients:

1 head Boston lettuce, rinsed, patted and shredded

½ cup capers

½ cup artichoke hearts

Dressing

2 tbsp. red wine vinegar

4 tablespoons extra virgin olive oil

Freshly ground black pepper

3/4 cup finely ground almonds

Sea salt

Prep

Combine all of the dressing ingredients in a food processor.

Toss with the rest of the ingredients and combine well.

Romaine Lettuce Green Olives and Artichoke Heart with Macadamia Vinaigrette

Ingredients:

1 head romaine lettuce, rinsed, patted and shredded

½ cup green olives

½ cup artichoke hearts

Dressing

2 tbsp. balsamic vinegar

4 tablespoons macadamia oil

Freshly ground black pepper

3/4 cup finely coarsely ground cashews

Sea salt

Prep

Combine all of the dressing ingredients in a food processor.

Toss with the rest of the ingredients and combine well.

Bib Lettuce Olive and Baby Carrot with Walnut Vinaigrette Salad

Ingredients:

1 head bib lettuce, rinsed, patted and shredded

½ cup black olives

½ cup baby carrots

Dressing

2 tbsp. apple cider vinegar

4 tablespoons extra virgin olive oil

Freshly ground black pepper

3/4 cup finely coarsely ground walnuts

Sea salt

Prep

Combine all of the dressing ingredients in a food processor.

Toss with the rest of the ingredients and combine well.

Romaine Lettuce with Baby Corn Salad

Ingredients:

1 head romaine lettuce, rinsed, patted and shredded

½ cup black olives

½ cup canned baby corn

Dressing

2 tbsp. red wine vinegar

4 tablespoons extra virgin olive oil

Freshly ground black pepper

3/4 cup finely ground almonds

Sea salt

Prep

Combine all of the dressing ingredients in a food processor.

Toss with the rest of the ingredients and combine well.

Romaine Lettuce Red Onion and Artichoke Heart with Peanut Vinaigrette Salad

Ingredients:

1 head romaine lettuce, rinsed, patted and shredded

½ cup chopped red onion

½ cup artichoke hearts

Dressing

2 tbsp. white wine vinegar

4 tablespoons extra virgin olive oil

Freshly ground black pepper

3/4 cup finely ground peanuts

Sea salt

Prep

Combine all of the dressing ingredients in a food processor.

Toss with the rest of the ingredients and combine well.

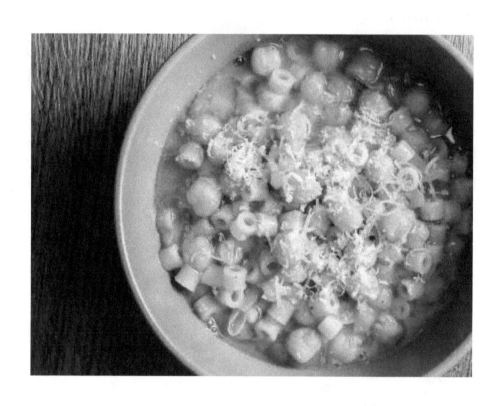

Boston Lettuce Black Olives and Baby Corn with Almond Vinaigrette Salad

Ingredients:

1 head Boston lettuce, rinsed, patted and shredded

½ cup black olives

½ cup canned baby corn

Dressing

2 tbsp. white wine vinegar

4 tablespoons olive oil

Freshly ground black pepper

3/4 cup finely ground almonds

Sea salt

Prep

Combine all of the dressing ingredients in a food processor.

Toss with the rest of the ingredients and combine well.

Endive and Green Olive Salad

Ingredients:

1 endives rinsed, patted and shredded

½ cup green olives

½ cup artichoke hearts

Dressing

2 tbsp. white wine vinegar

4 tablespoons macadamia oil

Freshly ground black pepper

3/4 cup finely coarsely ground cashews

Sea salt

Prep

Combine all of the dressing ingredients in a food processor.

Toss with the rest of the ingredients and combine well.

Mixed Greens Olives and Artichoke Heart Salad

Ingredients:

1 bunch of mixed greens, rinsed, patted and shredded

½ cup black olives

½ cup artichoke hearts

Dressing

2 tbsp. white wine vinegar

4 tablespoons extra virgin olive oil

Freshly ground black pepper

3/4 cup finely coarsely ground walnuts

Sea salt

Prep

Combine all of the dressing ingredients in a food processor.

Toss with the rest of the ingredients and combine well.

Boston Lettuce and Artichoke Heart Salad

Ingredients:

1 head Boston lettuce, rinsed, patted and shredded

½ cup Kalamata olives

½ cup artichoke hearts

Dressing

2 tbsp. balsamic vinegar

4 tablespoons extra virgin olive oil

Freshly ground black pepper

3/4 cup finely ground almonds

Sea salt

Prep

Combine all of the dressing ingredients in a food processor.

Toss with the rest of the ingredients and combine well.

Grilled Asparagus Green Pepper and Squash

Marinade Ingredients

1/4 cup extra virgin olive oil

2 tablespoons honey

4 teaspoons balsamic vinegar

1 teaspoon dried oregano

1 teaspoon garlic powder

1/8 teaspoon rainbow peppercorns

Sea salt

Vegetable Ingredients

1 pound fresh asparagus, trimmed

3 small carrots, cut in half lengthwise

1 large sweet green pepper, cut into 1-inch strips

1 medium yellow summer squash, cut into 1/2-inch slices

1 medium yellow onion, cut into wedges

Combine the marinade ingredients.

Combine the 3 tablespoons marinade and vegetables in a bag.

Marinate 1 1/2 hours at room temperature or overnight in the refrigerator.

Grill the vegetables over medium heat for 8-12 minutes or until tender.

Sprinkle the remaining marinade.

Simple Grilled Zucchini and Red Onions

Ingredients

2 large zucchini , cut lengthwise into ½ inch slabs

2 large red onions, cut into ½ inch rings but don't separate into individual rings

2 tbsp. extra virgin olive oil

2 tbsp. ranch dressing mix

Lightly brush each side of the vegetables with olive oil.

Season with the ranch dressing mix

Grill over 4 minutes over medium heat or until tender.

Simple Grilled Corns and Portobello

Ingredients

2 large Corn, cut lengthwise

5 pcs. Portobello, rinsed and drained

Marinade Ingredients:

6 tbsp. extra virgin olive oil

Sea salt, to taste

3 tbsp. distilled white vinegar

1 tsp. Dijon mustard

Marinate the vegetable with the dressing or marinade ingredients for 15 to 30 min.

Grill for 4 minutes over medium heat or until the vegetable becomes tender.

Grilled Marinated Eggplant and Zucchini

Ingredients

2 large Eggplants, cut lengthwise and cut in half

2 large Zucchinis, cut lengthwise and cut in half

Marinade Ingredients:

6 tbsp. extra virgin olive oil

Sea salt, to taste

3 tbsp. distilled white vinegar

1 tsp. Dijon mustard

Marinate the vegetable with the dressing or marinade ingredients for 15 to 30 min.

Grill for 4 minutes over medium heat or until the vegetable becomes tender.

Grilled Bell Pepper and Broccolini

Ingredients

2 Green Bell Peppers, cut in half

10 Broccolini Florets

Marinade Ingredients:

6 tbsp. extra virgin olive oil

Sea salt, to taste

3 tbsp. distilled white vinegar

1 tsp. Dijon mustard

Marinate the vegetable with the dressing or marinade ingredients for 15 to 30 min.

Grill for 4 minutes over medium heat or until the vegetable becomes tender.

Grilled Cauliflower and Brussel Sprouts

Ingredients

10 Cauliflower florets

10 pcs. Brussel Sprouts

Marinade Ingredients:

6 tbsp. extra virgin olive oil

Sea salt, to taste

3 tbsp. distilled white vinegar

1 tsp. Dijon mustard

Marinate the vegetable with the dressing or marinade ingredients for 15 to 30 min.

Grill for 4 minutes over medium heat or until the vegetable becomes tender.

Grilled Corn and Crimini Mushrooms

Ingredients

2 Corns, cut lengthwise

10 Crimini Mushrooms, rinsed and drained

Marinade Ingredients:

6 tbsp. extra virgin olive oil

Sea salt, to taste

3 tbsp. distilled white vinegar

1 tsp. Dijon mustard

Marinate the vegetable with the dressing or marinade ingredients for 15 to 30 min.

Grill for 4 minutes over medium heat or until the vegetable becomes tender.

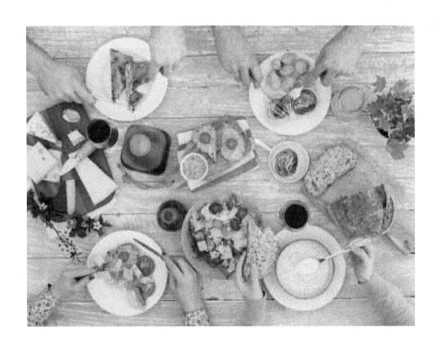

Grilled Eggplant, Zucchini and Corn

Ingredients

2 large Eggplants, cut lengthwise and cut in half

2 large Zucchinis, cut lengthwise and cut in half

2 Corns, cut lengthwise

Marinade Ingredients:

6 tbsp. extra virgin olive oil

Sea salt, to taste

3 tbsp. distilled white vinegar

1 tsp. Dijon mustard

Marinate the vegetable with the dressing or marinade ingredients for 15 to 30 min.

Grill for 4 minutes over medium heat or until the vegetable becomes tender.

Grilled Zucchini and Pineapple

Ingredients

2 large zucchini , cut lengthwise into ½ inch slabs

2 large red onions, cut into ½ inch rings but don't separate into individual rings

1 medium Pineapple, cut into 1/2 inch slices

10 Green Beans

Marinade Ingredients:

6 tbsp. extra virgin olive oil

Sea salt, to taste

3 tbsp. distilled white vinegar

1 tsp. Dijon mustard

Marinate the vegetable with the dressing or marinade ingredients for 15 to 30 min.

Grill for 4 minutes over medium heat or until the vegetable becomes tender.

Grilled Portobello and Asparagus

Ingredients

3 pcs. Portobello, rinsed and drained

2 pcs. Eggplant, cut lengthwise and cut in half

2 pcs. Zucchini, cut lengthwise and cut in half

6 pcs. Asparagus

Marinade Ingredients:

6 tbsp. extra virgin olive oil

Sea salt, to taste

3 tbsp. distilled white vinegar

1 tsp. Dijon mustard

Marinate the vegetable with the dressing or marinade ingredients for 15 to 30 min.

Grill for 4 minutes over medium heat or until the vegetable becomes tender.

Simple Grilled Vegetables Recipe

Ingredients

3 pcs. Portobello, rinsed and drained

2 pcs. Eggplant, cut lengthwise and cut in half

2 pcs. Zucchini, cut lengthwise and cut in half

6 pcs. Asparagus

Dressing Ingredients

6 tbsp. extra virgin olive oil

Sea salt, to taste

3 tbsp. apple cider vinegar

1 tbsp. honey

1 tsp. Egg-free mayonnaise

Marinate the vegetable with the dressing or marinade ingredients for 15 to 30 min.

Grill for 4 minutes over medium heat or until the vegetable becomes tender.

Grilled Japanese Eggplant and Shitake Mushroom

Ingredients

Corns, cut lengthwise

2 pcs. Japanese Eggplant, cut lengthwise and cut in half

Shitake Mushroom, rinsed and drained

Dressing Ingredients

6 tbsp. olive oil

Sea salt, to taste

3 tbsp. white wine vinegar

1 tsp. Egg-free mayonnaise

Marinate the vegetable with the dressing or marinade ingredients for 15 to 30 min.

Grill for 4 minutes over medium heat or until the vegetable becomes tender.

Grilled Japanese Eggplant and Broccolini

Ingredients

2 Green Bell Peppers, cut in half

10 Broccolini Florets

2 pcs. Japanese Eggplant, cut lengthwise and cut in half

Dressing Ingredients

6 tbsp. sesame oil

Sea salt, to taste

3 tbsp. distilled white vinegar

1 tsp. Egg-free mayonnaise

Marinate the vegetable with the dressing or marinade ingredients for 15 to 30 min.

Grill for 4 minutes over medium heat or until the vegetable becomes tender.

Grilled Cauliflower and Brussel Sprouts

Ingredients

10 Cauliflower florets

10 pcs. Brussel Sprouts

Dressing Ingredients

6 tbsp. sesame oil

Sea salt, to taste

3 tbsp. distilled white vinegar

1 tsp. Egg-free mayonnaise

Marinate the vegetable with the dressing or marinade ingredients for 15 to 30 min.

Grill for 4 minutes over medium heat or until the vegetable becomes tender.

Grilled Japanese and Cauliflower Recipe with Balsamic Glaze

Ingredients

2 Green Bell Peppers, cut in half lengthwise

10 Cauliflower Florets

2 pcs. Japanese Eggplant, cut lengthwise and cut in half

Dressing Ingredients

6 tbsp. extra virgin olive oil

Sea salt, to taste

3 tbsp. Balsamic vinegar

1 tsp. Dijon mustard

Marinate the vegetable with the dressing or marinade ingredients for 15 to 30 min.

Grill for 4 minutes over medium heat or until the vegetable becomes tender.

Simple Grilled Vegetables Recipe

Ingredients

2 large Eggplants, cut lengthwise and cut in half

1 large Zucchini, cut lengthwise and cut in half

5 Broccoli Florets

Marinade Ingredients:

6 tbsp. extra virgin olive oil

Sea salt, to taste

3 tbsp. distilled white vinegar

1 tsp. Dijon mustard

Marinate the vegetable with the dressing or marinade ingredients for 15 to 30 min.

Grill for 4 minutes over medium heat or until the vegetable becomes tender.

Grilled Eggplant and Green Bell Peppers

Ingredients

2 Green Bell Peppers, cut in half

10 Broccolini Florets

2 pcs. Eggplant, cut lengthwise and cut in half

Dressing Ingredients

6 tbsp. olive oil

Sea salt, to taste

3 tbsp. white wine vinegar

1 tsp. English mustard

Marinate the vegetable with the dressing or marinade ingredients for 15 to 30 min.

Grill for 4 minutes over medium heat or until the vegetable becomes tender.

Grilled Portobello Asparagus and Green Beans with Apple Cider Vinaigrette

Ingredients

3 pcs. Portobello, rinsed and drained

2 pcs. Eggplant, cut lengthwise and cut in half

2 pcs. Zucchini, cut lengthwise and cut in half

6 pcs. Asparagus

1 medium Pineapple, cut into 1/2 inch slices

10 Green Beans

Dressing Ingredients

6 tbsp. extra virgin olive oil

Sea salt, to taste

3 tbsp. apple cider vinegar

1 tbsp. honey

1 tsp. Egg-free mayonnaise

Marinate the vegetable with the dressing or marinade ingredients for 15 to 30 min.

Grill for 4 minutes over medium heat or until the vegetable becomes tender.

Grilled Beans and Portobello Mushrooms

Ingredients

Corns, cut lengthwise

5 pcs. Portobello mushrooms, rinsed and drained

10 Green Beans

Dressing Ingredients

6 tbsp. olive oil

Sea salt, to taste

3 tbsp. white wine vinegar

1 tsp. Egg-free mayonnaise

Marinate the vegetable with the dressing or marinade ingredients for 15 to 30 min.

Grill for 4 minutes over medium heat or until the vegetable becomes tender.

Brussel Sprouts and Green Beans

Ingredients

10 Cauliflower florets

10 pcs. Brussel Sprouts

10 Green Beans

Dressing Ingredients

6 tbsp. olive oil

Sea salt, to taste

3 tbsp. white wine vinegar

1 tsp. Egg-free mayonnaise

Marinate the vegetable with the dressing or marinade ingredients for 15 to 30 min.

Grill for 4 minutes over medium heat or until the vegetable becomes tender.

Zucchini and Onion in Ranch Dressing

Ingredients

2 large zucchini , cut lengthwise into ½ inch slabs

2 large red onions, cut into ½ inch rings but don't separate into individual rings

2 tbsp. extra virgin olive oil

2 tbsp. ranch dressing mix

Marinate the vegetable with the dressing or marinade ingredients for 15 to 30 min.

Grill for 4 minutes over medium heat or until the vegetable becomes tender.

Grilled Green Bean and Pineapple in Balsamic Vinaigrette

Ingredients

1 medium Pineapple, cut into 1/2 inch slices

10 Green Beans

Dressing Ingredients

6 tbsp. extra virgin olive oil

Sea salt, to taste

3 tbsp. Balsamic vinegar

1 tsp. Dijon mustard

Marinate the vegetable with the dressing or marinade ingredients for 15 to 30 min.

Grill for 4 minutes over medium heat or until the vegetable becomes tender.

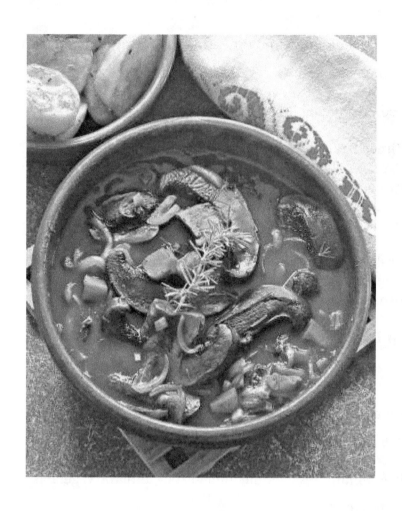

Grilled Broccolini and Eggplants

Ingredients

1 large Eggplants, cut lengthwise and cut in half

1 large Zucchinis, cut lengthwise and cut in half

10 Green Beans

10 Broccolini Florets

Marinade Ingredients:

6 tbsp. extra virgin olive oil

Sea salt, to taste

3 tbsp. distilled white vinegar

1 tsp. Dijon mustard

Marinate the vegetable with the dressing or marinade ingredients for 15 to 30 min.

Grill for 4 minutes over medium heat or until the vegetable becomes tender.

Grilled Broccolini and Green Bell Peppers

Ingredients

2 Green Bell Peppers, cut in half

8 Broccolini Florets

Dressing Ingredients

6 tbsp. sesame oil

Sea salt, to taste

3 tbsp. distilled white vinegar

1 tsp. Egg-free mayonnaise

Marinate the vegetable with the dressing or marinade ingredients for 15 to 30 min.

Grill for 4 minutes over medium heat or until the vegetable becomes tender.

Grilled Zucchini and Carrots

Ingredients

2 large zucchini , cut lengthwise into ½ inch slabs

1 large red onion, cut into ½ inch rings but don't separate into individual rings

1 large carrot, peeled and cut lengthwise

Dressing Ingredients

6 tbsp. olive oil

Sea salt, to taste

3 tbsp. white wine vinegar

1 tsp. English mustard

Marinate the vegetable with the dressing or marinade ingredients for 15 to 30 min.

Grill for 4 minutes over medium heat or until the vegetable becomes tender.

Grilled Portobello Mushrooms in Apple Cider Vinaigrette

Ingredients

Corns, cut lengthwise

5 pcs. Portobello mushrooms, rinsed and drained

Dressing Ingredients

6 tbsp. extra virgin olive oil

Sea salt, to taste

3 tbsp. apple cider vinegar

1 tbsp. honey

1 tsp. Egg-free mayonnaise

Marinate the vegetable with the dressing or marinade ingredients for 15 to 30 min.

Grill for 4 minutes over medium heat or until the vegetable becomes tender.

Grilled Carrots with Brussel Sprouts

Ingredients

10 Cauliflower florets

10 pcs. Brussel Sprouts

1 large carrot, peeled and cut lengthwise

Dressing Ingredients

6 tbsp. olive oil

Sea salt, to taste

3 tbsp. white wine vinegar

1 tsp. Egg-free mayonnaise

Marinate the vegetable with the dressing or marinade ingredients for 15 to 30 min.

Grill for 4 minutes over medium heat or until the vegetable becomes tender.

Grilled Parsnip and Zucchini Recipe

Ingredients

1 large parsnip, peeled and cut lengthwise

1 large zucchini , cut lengthwise into ½ inch slabs

2 large red onions, cut into ½ inch rings but don't separate into individual rings

Marinade Ingredients:

6 tbsp. extra virgin olive oil

Sea salt, to taste

3 tbsp. distilled white vinegar

1 tsp. Dijon mustard

Marinate the vegetable with the dressing or marinade ingredients for 15 to 30 min.

Grill for 4 minutes over medium heat or until the vegetable becomes tender.

Grilled Turnip in Oriental Vinaigrette

Ingredients

1 large turnip, peeled and cut lengthwise

2 Green Bell Peppers, cut in half

10 Broccolini Florets

Dressing Ingredients

6 tbsp. sesame oil

Sea salt, to taste

3 tbsp. distilled white vinegar

1 tsp. Egg-free mayonnaise

Marinate the vegetable with the dressing or marinade ingredients for 15 to 30 min.

Grill for 4 minutes over medium heat or until the vegetable becomes tender.

Grilled Carrot, Turnip and Portobello with Balsamic Glaze

Ingredients

1 large carrots, peeled and cut lengthwise

1 large turnip, peeled and cut lengthwise

1 Corn, cut lengthwise

2 pcs. Portobello mushrooms, rinsed and drained

Dressing Ingredients

6 tbsp. extra virgin olive oil

Sea salt, to taste

3 tbsp. Balsamic vinegar

1 tsp. Dijon mustard

Marinate the vegetable with the dressing or marinade ingredients for 15 to 30 min.

Grill for 4 minutes over medium heat or until the vegetable becomes tender.

Grilled Zucchinis and Mangoes

Ingredients

2 large Zucchinis, cut lengthwise and cut in half

2 large mangoes, cut lengthwise and pitted

Dressing Ingredients

6 tbsp. sesame oil

Sea salt, to taste

3 tbsp. distilled white vinegar

1 tsp. Egg-free mayonnaise

Marinate the vegetable with the dressing or marinade ingredients for 15 to 30 min.

Grill for 4 minutes over medium heat or until the vegetable becomes tender.

For the mango, grill only until you start seeing brown grill marks.

Grilled Baby Corn and Green Beans

Ingredients

½ cup baby corn

1 medium Pineapple, cut into 1/2 inch slices

10 Green Beans

2 large red onions, cut into ½ inch rings but don't separate into individual rings

Dressing Ingredients

6 tbsp. olive oil

Sea salt, to taste

3 tbsp. white wine vinegar

1 tsp. English mustard

Marinate the vegetable with the dressing or marinade ingredients for 15 to 30 min.

Grill for 4 minutes over medium heat or until the vegetable becomes tender.

Grilled Artichoke Hearts and Brussel Sprouts

Ingredients

½ cup canned artichoke hearts

5 Broccoli Florets

10 pcs. Brussel Sprouts

Dressing Ingredients

6 tbsp. olive oil

Sea salt, to taste

3 tbsp. white wine vinegar

1 tsp. Egg-free mayonnaise

Marinate the vegetable with the dressing or marinade ingredients for 15 to 30 min.

Grill for 4 minutes over medium heat or until the vegetable becomes tender.

Grilles Bell Peppers Broccolini and Brussel Sprouts with Honey Apple Cider Glaze

Ingredients

10 Broccolini Florets

½ cup canned artichoke hearts

10 Brussel Sprouts

Dressing Ingredients

6 tbsp. extra virgin olive oil

Sea salt, to taste

3 tbsp. apple cider vinegar

1 tbsp. honey

1 tsp. Egg-free mayonnaise

Marinate the vegetable with the dressing or marinade ingredients for 15 to 30 min.

Grill for 4 minutes over medium heat or until the vegetable becomes tender.

Grilled Assorted Bell Peppers with Broccolini Florets Recipe

Ingredients

1 Green Bell Pepper, cut in half

1 Yellow Bell Pepper, cut in half

1 Red Bell Pepper, cut in half

10 Broccolini Florets

Marinade Ingredients:

6 tbsp. extra virgin olive oil

Sea salt, to taste

3 tbsp. distilled white vinegar

1 tsp. Dijon mustard

Marinate the vegetable with the dressing or marinade ingredients for 15 to 30 min.

Grill for 4 minutes over medium heat or until the vegetable becomes tender.

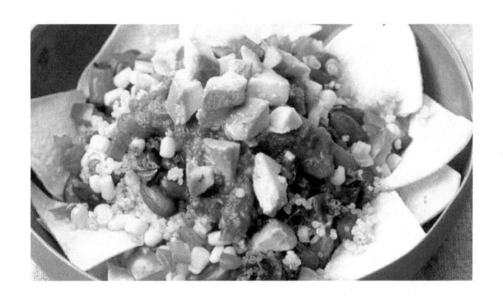

Grilled Eggplant, Zucchini with Assorted Bell Peppers

Ingredients

1 small Eggplant, cut lengthwise and cut in half

1 small Zucchini, cut lengthwise and cut in half

1 Green Bell Pepper, cut in half

1 Yellow Bell Pepper, cut in half

1 Red Bell Pepper, cut in half

Dressing Ingredients

6 tbsp. sesame oil

Sea salt, to taste

3 tbsp. distilled white vinegar

1 tsp. Egg-free mayonnaise

Marinate the vegetable with the dressing or marinade ingredients for 15 to 30 min.

Grill for 4 minutes over medium heat or until the vegetable becomes tender.

Grilled Portobello and Red Onion

Ingredients

1 Corn, cut lengthwise

5 pcs. Portobello mushrooms, rinsed and drained

1 medium red onion, cut into ½ inch rings but don't separate into individual rings

Dressing Ingredients

6 tbsp. extra virgin olive oil

Sea salt, to taste

3 tbsp. Balsamic vinegar

1 tsp. Dijon mustard

Marinate the vegetable with the dressing or marinade ingredients for 15 to 30 min.

Grill for 4 minutes over medium heat or until the vegetable becomes tender.

Grilled Corn and Red Onions

Ingredients

2 large zucchini , cut lengthwise into ½ inch slabs

2 large red onions, cut into ½ inch rings but don't separate into individual rings

1 Corn, cut Lengthwise

Dressing Ingredients

6 tbsp. sesame oil

Sea salt, to taste

3 tbsp. distilled white vinegar

1 tsp. Egg-free mayonnaise

Marinate the vegetable with the dressing or marinade ingredients for 15 to 30 min.

Grill for 4 minutes over medium heat or until the vegetable becomes tender.

Grilled Brussel Sprouts Cauliflower and Asparagus

Ingredients

10 Cauliflower florets

5 pcs. Brussel Sprouts

6 pcs. Asparagus

Dressing Ingredients

6 tbsp. olive oil

Sea salt, to taste

3 tbsp. white wine vinegar

1 tsp. English mustard

Marinate the vegetable with the dressing or marinade ingredients for 15 to 30 min.

Grill for 4 minutes over medium heat or until the vegetable becomes tender.

Grilled Zucchini Eggplants Portobello and Asparagus

Ingredients

3 pcs. Portobello, rinsed and drained

2 pcs. Eggplant, cut lengthwise and cut in half

2 pcs. Zucchini, cut lengthwise and cut in half

6 pcs. Asparagus

Dressing Ingredients

6 tbsp. sesame oil

Sea salt, to taste

3 tbsp. distilled white vinegar

1 tsp. Egg-free mayonnaise

Marinate the vegetable with the dressing or marinade ingredients for 15 to 30 min.

Grill for 4 minutes over medium heat or until the vegetable becomes tender.

Grilled Green Bell Pepper, Broccolini and Asparagus Recipe

Ingredients

2 Green Bell Peppers, cut in half

5 Broccolini Florets

6 pcs. Asparagus

Dressing Ingredients

6 tbsp. extra virgin olive oil

Sea salt, to taste

3 tbsp. apple cider vinegar

1 tbsp. honey

1 tsp. Egg-free mayonnaise

Marinate the vegetable with the dressing or marinade ingredients for 15 to 30 min.

Grill for 4 minutes over medium heat or until the vegetable becomes tender.

Grilled Portobello Mushroom and Zucchini

Ingredients

2 large zucchini , cut lengthwise into ½ inch slabs

2 large red onions, cut into ½ inch rings but don't separate into individual rings

2 Portobello mushroom, cut in half

Marinade Ingredients:

6 tbsp. extra virgin olive oil

Sea salt, to taste

3 tbsp. distilled white vinegar

1 tsp. Dijon mustard

Marinate the vegetable with the dressing or marinade ingredients for 15 to 30 min.

Grill for 4 minutes over medium heat or until the vegetable becomes tender.

Grilled Asparagus Pineapple and Green Beans

Ingredients

10 Broccolini Florets

10 pcs. Asparagus

1 medium Pineapple, cut into 1/2 inch slices

10 Green Beans

Dressing Ingredients

6 tbsp. sesame oil

Sea salt, to taste

3 tbsp. distilled white vinegar

1 tsp. Egg-free mayonnaise

Marinate the vegetable with the dressing or marinade ingredients for 15 to 30 min.

Grill for 4 minutes over medium heat or until the vegetable becomes tender.

Grilled Green Beans and Eggplants

Ingredients

2 large Eggplants, cut lengthwise and cut in half

2 large Zucchinis, cut lengthwise and cut in half

10 Green Beans

Dressing Ingredients

6 tbsp. extra virgin olive oil

Sea salt, to taste

3 tbsp. Balsamic vinegar

1 tsp. Dijon mustard

Marinate the vegetable with the dressing or marinade ingredients for 15 to 30 min.

Grill for 4 minutes over medium heat or until the vegetable becomes tender.

Grilled Asparagus and Broccolini

Ingredients

Corns, cut lengthwise

5 pcs. Portobello mushrooms, rinsed and drained

8 pcs. Asparagus

Dressing Ingredients

6 tbsp. sesame oil

Sea salt, to taste

3 tbsp. distilled white vinegar

1 tsp. Egg-free mayonnaise

Marinate the vegetable with the dressing or marinade ingredients for 15 to 30 min.

Grill for 4 minutes over medium heat or until the vegetable becomes tender.

Grilled Cauliflower and Brussel Sprouts

Ingredients

10 Cauliflower florets

10 pcs. Brussel Sprouts

10 Broccolini Florets

10 pcs. Asparagus

Dressing Ingredients

6 tbsp. olive oil

Sea salt, to taste

3 tbsp. white wine vinegar

1 tsp. English mustard

Marinate the vegetable with the dressing or marinade ingredients for 15 to 30 min.

Grill for 4 minutes over medium heat or until the vegetable becomes tender.

Grilled Broccoli and Broccolini Florets

Ingredients

2 Green Bell Peppers, cut in half

5 Broccolini Florets

5 Broccoli Florets

Dressing Ingredients

6 tbsp. sesame oil

Sea salt, to taste

3 tbsp. distilled white vinegar

1 tsp. Egg-free mayonnaise

Marinate the vegetable with the dressing or marinade ingredients for 15 to 30 min.

Grill for 4 minutes over medium heat or until the vegetable becomes tender.

Grilled Zucchini Red Onions Broccolini Florets and Asparagus

Ingredients

2 large zucchini , cut lengthwise into ½ inch slabs

2 large red onions, cut into ½ inch rings but don't separate into individual rings

10 Broccolini Florets

10 pcs. Asparagus

Dressing Ingredients

6 tbsp. extra virgin olive oil

Sea salt, to taste

3 tbsp. apple cider vinegar

1 tbsp. honey

1 tsp. Egg-free mayonnaise

Marinate the vegetable with the dressing or marinade ingredients for 15 to 30 min.

Grill for 4 minutes over medium heat or until the vegetable becomes tender.

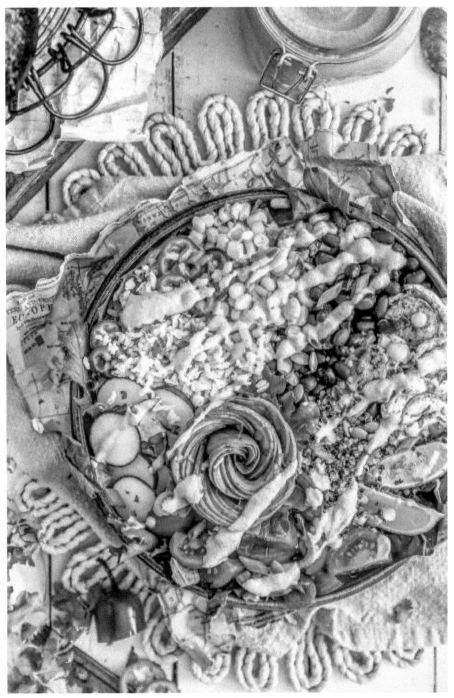

Grilled Green Beans Asparagus Broccolini Florets and Pineapple

Ingredients

10 Broccolini Florets

10 pcs. Asparagus

1 medium Pineapple, cut into 1/2 inch slices

10 Green Beans

Marinade Ingredients:

6 tbsp. extra virgin olive oil

Sea salt, to taste

3 tbsp. distilled white vinegar

1 tsp. Dijon mustard

Marinate the vegetable with the dressing or marinade ingredients for 15 to 30 min.

Grill for 4 minutes over medium heat or until the vegetable becomes tender.

Grilled Edamame Beans

Ingredients

10 Edamame Beans

10 Cauliflower florets

10 pcs. Brussel Sprouts

Dressing Ingredients

6 tbsp. olive oil

Sea salt, to taste

3 tbsp. white wine vinegar

1 tsp. Egg-free mayonnaise

Marinate the vegetable with the dressing or marinade ingredients for 15 to 30 min.

Grill for 4 minutes over medium heat or until the vegetable becomes tender.

Grilled Okra, Zucchini and Red Onions

Ingredients

5 pcs. Okra

2 large zucchini , cut lengthwise into ½ inch slabs

2 large red onions, cut into ½ inch rings but don't separate into individual rings

Dressing Ingredients

6 tbsp. extra virgin olive oil

Sea salt, to taste

3 tbsp. Balsamic vinegar

1 tsp. Dijon mustard

Marinate the vegetable with the dressing or marinade ingredients for 15 to 30 min.

Grill for 4 minutes over medium heat or until the vegetable becomes tender.

Grilled Parsnip and Zucchini

Ingredients

1 large Parsnip, cut lengthwise

2 large zucchini , cut lengthwise into ½ inch slabs

2 large red onions, cut into ½ inch rings but don't separate into individual rings

2 tbsp. extra virgin olive oil

2 tbsp. ranch dressing mix

Marinate the vegetable with the dressing or marinade ingredients for 15 to 30 min.

Grill for 4 minutes over medium heat or until the vegetable becomes tender.

Grilled Parsnip and Okra

Ingredients

1 large Parsnip, cut lengthwise

5 pcs. Okra

2 large Eggplants, cut lengthwise and cut in half

2 large Zucchinis, cut lengthwise and cut in half

Dressing Ingredients

6 tbsp. olive oil

Sea salt, to taste

3 tbsp. white wine vinegar

1 tsp. English mustard

Marinate the vegetable with the dressing or marinade ingredients for 15 to 30 min.

Grill for 4 minutes over medium heat or until the vegetable becomes tender.

Grilled Broccoli Parsnip Okra and Asparagus

Ingredients

5 Broccolini Florets

1 large Parsnip, cut lengthwise

5 pcs. Okra

3 pcs. Asparagus

Corns, cut lengthwise

2 pcs. Portobello mushrooms, rinsed and drained

Marinade Ingredients:

6 tbsp. extra virgin olive oil

Sea salt, to taste

3 tbsp. distilled white vinegar

1 tsp. Dijon mustard

Marinate the vegetable with the dressing or marinade ingredients for 15 to 30 min.

Grill for 4 minutes over medium heat or until the vegetable becomes tender.

Grilled Turnip and Bell Peppers

Ingredients

1 large Turnip, cut lengthwise

2 Green Bell Peppers, cut in half

10 Broccolini Florets

Dressing Ingredients

6 tbsp. extra virgin olive oil

Sea salt, to taste

3 tbsp. apple cider vinegar

1 tbsp. honey

1 tsp. Egg-free mayonnaise

Marinate the vegetable with the dressing or marinade ingredients for 15 to 30 min.

Grill for 4 minutes over medium heat or until the vegetable becomes tender.

Grilled Cauliflower and Broccolini

Ingredients

10 Cauliflower florets

10 pcs. Brussel Sprouts

10 Broccolini Florets

10 pcs. Asparagus

Dressing Ingredients

6 tbsp. sesame oil

Sea salt, to taste

3 tbsp. distilled white vinegar

1 tsp. Egg-free mayonnaise

Marinate the vegetable with the dressing or marinade ingredients for 15 to 30 min.

Grill for 4 minutes over medium heat or until the vegetable becomes tender.

Grilled Turnip and Pineapple

Ingredients

1 large Turnip, cut lengthwise

1 medium Pineapple, cut into 1/2 inch slices

10 Green Beans

Dressing Ingredients

6 tbsp. sesame oil

Sea salt, to taste

3 tbsp. distilled white vinegar

1 tsp. Egg-free mayonnaise

Marinate the vegetable with the dressing or marinade ingredients for 15 to 30 min.

Grill for 4 minutes over medium heat or until the vegetable becomes tender.

Grilled Parsnip and Zucchini

Ingredients

1 large Parsnip, cut lengthwise

2 large zucchini , cut lengthwise into ½ inch slabs

2 large red onions, cut into ½ inch rings but don't separate into individual rings

Dressing Ingredients

6 tbsp. olive oil

Sea salt, to taste

3 tbsp. white wine vinegar

1 tsp. Egg-free mayonnaise

Marinate the vegetable with the dressing or marinade ingredients for 15 to 30 min.

Grill for 4 minutes over medium heat or until the vegetable becomes tender.

Grilled Turnip Red Onions and Parsnip

Ingredients

1 large Turnip, cut lengthwise

1 large Parsnip, cut lengthwise

1 large zucchini , cut lengthwise into ½ inch slabs

2 small red onions, cut into ½ inch rings but don't separate into individual rings

Dressing Ingredients

6 tbsp. extra virgin olive oil

Sea salt, to taste

3 tbsp. Balsamic vinegar

1 tsp. Dijon mustard

Marinate the vegetable with the dressing or marinade ingredients for 15 to 30 min.

Grill for 4 minutes over medium heat or until the vegetable becomes tender.

Grilled Carrot, Parsnip and Broccolini

Ingredients

1 large Carrot, cut lengthwise

1 large Parsnip, cut lengthwise

10 Broccolini Florets

10 pcs. Asparagus

10 Green Beans

Dressing Ingredients

6 tbsp. olive oil

Sea salt, to taste

3 tbsp. white wine vinegar

1 tsp. English mustard

Marinate the vegetable with the dressing or marinade ingredients for 15 to 30 min.

Grill for 4 minutes over medium heat or until the vegetable becomes tender.

Grilled Asparagus and Broccolini Florets

Ingredients

10 Broccolini Florets

10 pcs. Asparagus

Corns, cut lengthwise

5 pcs. Portobello mushrooms, rinsed and drained

Marinade Ingredients:

6 tbsp. extra virgin olive oil

Sea salt, to taste

3 tbsp. distilled white vinegar

1 tsp. Dijon mustard

Marinate the vegetable with the dressing or marinade ingredients for 15 to 30 min.

Grill for 4 minutes over medium heat or until the vegetable becomes tender.

Grilled Cauliflower and Baby Corn

Ingredients

10 Cauliflower florets

½ cup canned baby corn

10 pcs. Brussel Sprouts

Dressing Ingredients

6 tbsp. extra virgin olive oil

Sea salt, to taste

3 tbsp. apple cider vinegar

1 tbsp. honey

1 tsp. Egg-free mayonnaise

Marinate the vegetable with the dressing or marinade ingredients for 15 to 30 min.

Grill for 4 minutes over medium heat or until the vegetable becomes tender.

Grilled Artichoke Hearts and Broccolini Florets

Ingredients

½ cup canned artichoke hearts

10 Broccolini Florets

Dressing Ingredients

6 tbsp. sesame oil

Sea salt, to taste

3 tbsp. distilled white vinegar

1 tsp. Egg-free mayonnaise

Marinate the vegetable with the dressing or marinade ingredients for 15 to 30 min.

Grill for 4 minutes over medium heat or until the vegetable becomes tender.

Grilled Baby Carrots and Eggplants

Ingredients

5 pcs. baby carrots

2 large Eggplants, cut lengthwise and cut in half

2 large Zucchinis, cut lengthwise and cut in half

Dressing Ingredients

6 tbsp. sesame oil

Sea salt, to taste

3 tbsp. distilled white vinegar

1 tsp. Egg-free mayonnaise

Marinate the vegetable with the dressing or marinade ingredients for 15 to 30 min.

Grill for 4 minutes over medium heat or until the vegetable becomes tender.

Grilled Baby Carrots and Zucchini

Ingredients

7 pcs. baby carrots

2 large zucchini , cut lengthwise into ½ inch slabs

2 large red onions, cut into ½ inch rings but don't separate into individual rings

Dressing Ingredients

6 tbsp. olive oil

Sea salt, to taste

3 tbsp. white wine vinegar

1 tsp. Egg-free mayonnaise

Marinate the vegetable with the dressing or marinade ingredients for 15 to 30 min.

Grill for 4 minutes over medium heat or until the vegetable becomes tender.

Grilled Corn, Baby Corns and Asparagus

Ingredients

10 Baby Corns

10 pcs. Asparagus

Corns, cut lengthwise

Dressing Ingredients

6 tbsp. extra virgin olive oil

Sea salt, to taste

3 tbsp. Balsamic vinegar

1 tsp. Dijon mustard

Marinate the vegetable with the dressing or marinade ingredients for 15 to 30 min.

Grill for 4 minutes over medium heat or until the vegetable becomes tender.

Grilled Baby Carrots and Artichoke Hearts

Ingredients

1 cup canned artichoke hearts

2 large zucchini , cut lengthwise into ½ inch slabs

8 pcs. baby carrots

Dressing Ingredients

6 tbsp. olive oil

Sea salt, to taste

3 tbsp. white wine vinegar

1 tsp. English mustard

Marinate the vegetable with the dressing or marinade ingredients for 15 to 30 min.

Grill for 4 minutes over medium heat or until the vegetable becomes tender.

Grilled Pineapple Green Beans and Artichoke Hearts

Ingredients

1 medium Pineapple, cut into 1/2 inch slices

10 Green Beans

1 cup canned artichoke hearts

Marinade Ingredients:

6 tbsp. extra virgin olive oil

Sea salt, to taste

3 tbsp. distilled white vinegar

1 tsp. Dijon mustard

Marinate the vegetable with the dressing or marinade ingredients for 15 to 30 min.

Grill for 4 minutes over medium heat or until the vegetable becomes tender.

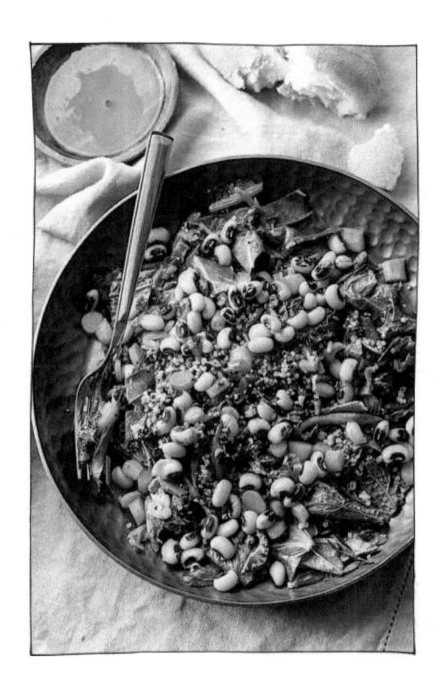

193

Grilled Broccolini and Baby Carrots

Ingredients

10 Broccolini Florets

10 pcs. Baby Carrots

2 large zucchini , cut lengthwise into ½ inch slabs

2 large red onions, cut into ½ inch rings but don't separate into individual rings

Dressing Ingredients

6 tbsp. olive oil

Sea salt, to taste

3 tbsp. white wine vinegar

1 tsp. Egg-free mayonnaise

Marinate the vegetable with the dressing or marinade ingredients for 15 to 30 min.

Grill for 4 minutes over medium heat or until the vegetable becomes tender.

Simple Grilled Baby Corn and Cauliflower Florets

Ingredients

10 pcs. Baby corn

10 Cauliflower florets

10 pcs. Brussel Sprouts

Dressing Ingredients

6 tbsp. extra virgin olive oil

Sea salt, to taste

3 tbsp. apple cider vinegar

1 tbsp. honey

1 tsp. Egg-free mayonnaise

Marinate the vegetable with the dressing or marinade ingredients for 15 to 30 min.

Grill for 4 minutes over medium heat or until the vegetable becomes tender.

Grilled Baby Carrots and Bell Peppers

Ingredients

8 pcs. baby carrots

2 Green Bell Peppers, cut in half

10 Broccolini Florets

Dressing Ingredients

6 tbsp. sesame oil

Sea salt, to taste

3 tbsp. distilled white vinegar

1 tsp. Egg-free mayonnaise

Marinate the vegetable with the dressing or marinade ingredients for 15 to 30 min.

Grill for 4 minutes over medium heat or until the vegetable becomes tender.

Grilled Baby Corn, Artichoke Hearts and Eggplant

Ingredients

½ cup canned baby corn

½ cup canned artichoke hearts

2 large Eggplants, cut lengthwise and cut in half

Dressing Ingredients

6 tbsp. olive oil

Sea salt, to taste

3 tbsp. white wine vinegar

1 tsp. Egg-free mayonnaise

Marinate the vegetable with the dressing or marinade ingredients for 15 to 30 min.

Grill for 4 minutes over medium heat or until the vegetable becomes tender.

Grilled Baby Carrots and Red Onion

Ingredients

½ cup baby carrots

2 large zucchini , cut lengthwise into ½ inch slabs

2 large red onions, cut into ½ inch rings but don't separate into individual rings

Dressing Ingredients

6 tbsp. extra virgin olive oil

Sea salt, to taste

3 tbsp. Balsamic vinegar

1 tsp. Dijon mustard

Marinate the vegetable with the dressing or marinade ingredients for 15 to 30 min.

Grill for 4 minutes over medium heat or until the vegetable becomes tender.

Grilled Broccolini Asparagus and Portobello Mushroom

Ingredients

10 Broccolini Florets

10 pcs. Asparagus

Corns, cut lengthwise

5 pcs. Portobello mushrooms, rinsed and drained

Dressing Ingredients

6 tbsp. sesame oil

Sea salt, to taste

3 tbsp. distilled white vinegar

1 tsp. Egg-free mayonnaise

Marinate the vegetable with the dressing or marinade ingredients for 15 to 30 min.

Grill for 4 minutes over medium heat or until the vegetable becomes tender.

Grilled Artichoke Hearts

Ingredients

1 cup canned artichoke hearts

2 large red onions, cut into ½ inch rings but don't separate into individual rings

Dressing Ingredients

6 tbsp. olive oil

Sea salt, to taste

3 tbsp. white wine vinegar

1 tsp. English mustard

Marinate the vegetable with the dressing or marinade ingredients for 15 to 30 min.

Grill for 4 minutes over medium heat or until the vegetable becomes tender.

Grilled Baby Carrots and Mushroom

Ingredients

10 pcs. Baby Carrots

1 cup canned button mushrooms

Dressing Ingredients

6 tbsp. olive oil

Sea salt, to taste

3 tbsp. white wine vinegar

1 tsp. Egg-free mayonnaise

Marinate the vegetable with the dressing or marinade ingredients for 15 to 30 min.

Grill for 4 minutes over medium heat or until the vegetable becomes tender.

Grilled Artichoke Hearts and Asparagus

Ingredients

½ cup canned artichoke hearts

10 Broccolini Florets

10 pcs. Asparagus

Dressing Ingredients

6 tbsp. extra virgin olive oil

Sea salt, to taste

3 tbsp. apple cider vinegar

1 tbsp. honey

1 tsp. Egg-free mayonnaise

Marinate the vegetable with the dressing or marinade ingredients for 15 to 30 min.

Grill for 4 minutes over medium heat or until the vegetable becomes tender.

Grilled Zucchini

Ingredients

2 large zucchini , cut lengthwise into ½ inch slabs

Dressing Ingredients

6 tbsp. olive oil

Sea salt, to taste

3 tbsp. white wine vinegar

1 tsp. Egg-free mayonnaise

Marinate the vegetable with the dressing or marinade ingredients for 15 to 30 min.

Grill for 4 minutes over medium heat or until the vegetable becomes tender.

Grilled Eggplant with Balsamic Glaze

Ingredients

2 large Eggplants, cut lengthwise and cut in half

Dressing Ingredients

6 tbsp. extra virgin olive oil

Sea salt, to taste

3 tbsp. Balsamic vinegar

1 tsp. Dijon mustard

Marinate the vegetable with the dressing or marinade ingredients for 15 to 30 min.

Grill for 4 minutes over medium heat or until the vegetable becomes tender.

Grilled Romaine Lettuce and Tomatoes

Ingredients

10 Broccolini Florets

10 pcs. Brussel Sprouts

10 pcs. Asparagus

1 bunch of Romaine Lettuce leaves

2 medium Carrots, cut lengthwise and cut in half

4 large Tomatoes, sliced thick

Dressing Ingredients:

6 tbsp. extra virgin olive oil

1 tsp. onion powder

Sea salt, to taste

3 tbsp. distilled white vinegar

1 tsp. Dijon mustard

Combine all of the dressing ingredients thoroughly.

Preheat your grill to low heat and grease the grates.

Layer the vegetables grill for 12 minutes per side, until tender flipping once.

Brush with the marinade/ dressing ingredients

Grilled Zucchini and Peppers

Ingredients

1 lb zucchini, sliced lengthwise into shorter sticks

1 lb green bell peppers, sliced into wide strips

1 large red onion, cut into 1/2 inch thick rounds

1/3 cup Italian parsley or basil, finely chopped

Dressing Ingredients

6 tbsp. olive oil

1 tsp. garlic powder

1 tsp. onion powder

Sea salt, to taste

3 tbsp. white wine vinegar

1 tsp. English mustard

Combine all of the dressing ingredients thoroughly.

Preheat your grill to low heat and grease the grates.

Layer the vegetables grill for 12 minutes per side, until tender flipping once.

Brush with the marinade/ dressing ingredients

Grilled Eggplant and Red Onion

Ingredients

1 lb eggplant, sliced lengthwise into shorter sticks

1 lb green bell peppers, sliced into wide strips

1 large red onion, cut into 1/2 inch thick rounds

1/3 cup Italian parsley or basil, finely chopped

Dressing Ingredients:

6 tbsp. extra virgin olive oil

1 tsp. onion powder

Sea salt, to taste

3 tbsp. distilled white vinegar

1 tsp. Dijon mustard

Combine all of the dressing ingredients thoroughly.

Preheat your grill to low heat and grease the grates.

Layer the vegetables grill for 12 minutes per side, until tender flipping once.

Brush with the marinade/ dressing ingredients

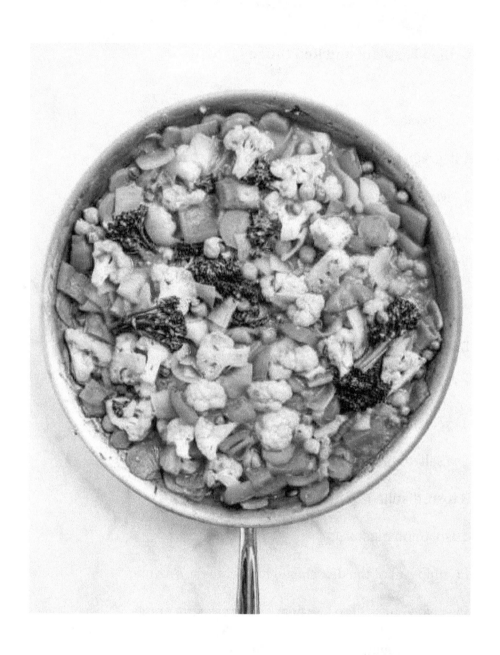

Grilled Asparagus Brussel Sprouts Broccolini Florets

Ingredients

10 pcs. Asparagus

1 bunch of Romaine Lettuce leaves

10 Broccolini Florets

10 pcs. Brussel Sprouts

2 medium Carrots, cut lengthwise and cut in half

4 large Tomatoes, sliced thick

Dressing Ingredients

6 tbsp. olive oil

3 dashes of Tabasco hot sauce

Sea salt, to taste

3 tbsp. white wine vinegar

1 tsp. Egg-free mayonnaise

Combine all of the dressing ingredients thoroughly.

Preheat your grill to low heat and grease the grates.

Layer the vegetables grill for 12 minutes per side, until tender flipping once.

Brush with the marinade/ dressing ingredients

Grilled Zucchini in Honey Apple Cider Glaze

Ingredients

1 lb zucchini, sliced lengthwise into shorter sticks

1 lb green bell peppers, sliced into wide strips

1 large red onion, cut into 1/2 inch thick rounds

1/3 cup Italian parsley or basil, finely chopped

Dressing Ingredients

6 tbsp. extra virgin olive oil

Sea salt, to taste

3 tbsp. apple cider vinegar

1 tbsp. honey

1 tsp. Egg-free mayonnaise

Combine all of the dressing ingredients thoroughly.

Preheat your grill to low heat and grease the grates.

Layer the vegetables grill for 12 minutes per side, until tender flipping once.

Brush with the marinade/ dressing ingredients

Grilled Zucchini Artichoke Hearts and Red Onion

Ingredients

1/2 lb zucchini, sliced lengthwise into shorter sticks

½ cup canned artichoke hearts

1 lb green bell peppers, sliced into wide strips

1 large red onion, cut into 1/2 inch thick rounds

1/3 cup Italian parsley or basil, finely chopped

Dressing Ingredients

6 tbsp. extra virgin olive oil

Sea salt, to taste

3 tbsp. Balsamic vinegar

1 tsp. Dijon mustard

Combine all of the dressing ingredients thoroughly.

Preheat your grill to low heat and grease the grates.

Layer the vegetables grill for 12 minutes per side, until tender flipping once.

Brush with the marinade/ dressing ingredients

Grilled Zucchini and Broccolini Florets

Ingredients

1 lb zucchini, sliced lengthwise into shorter sticks

1 lb green bell peppers, sliced into wide strips

10 Broccolini Florets

10 pcs. Brussel Sprouts

1 large red onion, cut into 1/2 inch thick rounds

1/3 cup Italian parsley or basil, finely chopped

Dressing Ingredients

6 tbsp. olive oil

1 tsp. garlic powder

1 tsp. onion powder

Sea salt, to taste

3 tbsp. white wine vinegar

1 tsp. English mustard

Combine all of the dressing ingredients thoroughly.

Preheat your grill to low heat and grease the grates.

Layer the vegetables grill for 12 minutes per side, until tender flipping once.

Brush with the marinade/ dressing ingredients

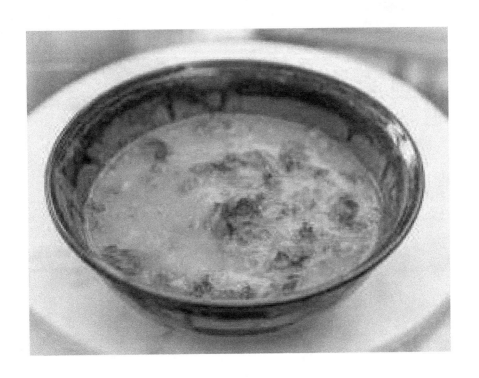

CPSIA information can be obtained
at www.ICGtesting.com
Printed in the USA
LVHW080731150622
721314LV00010B/698